OCT Angiography in Retinal and Macular Diseases

Developments in Ophthalmology

Vol. 56

Series Editor

F. Bandello Milan

OCT Angiography in Retinal and Macular Diseases

Volume Editors

Francesco Bandello Milan
Eric H. Souied Créteil
Giuseppe Querques Milan

120 figures, 107 in color, and 1 table, 2016

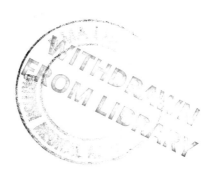

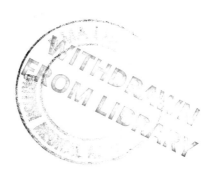

KARGER

Basel · Freiburg · Paris · London · New York · Chennai · New Delhi · Bangkok · Beijing · Shanghai · Tokyo · Kuala Lumpur · Singapore · Sydney

Francesco Bandello
Department of Ophthalmology
University Vita Salute
San Raffaele Scientific Institute
Via Olgettina, 60
IT–20132 Milan (Italy)

Giuseppe Querques
Head – Medical Retina & Imaging Unit
Department of Ophthalmology
University Vita Salute
San Raffaele Scientific Institute
Via Olgettina, 60
IT–20132 Milan (Italy)

Eric H. Souied
Department of Ophthalmology
Centre Hospitalier Intercommunal de Créteil
Universite Paris Est Créteil
40 Avenue de Verdun
FR–94000 Créteil (France)

Library of Congress Cataloging-in-Publication Data

Names: Bandello, F. (Francesco), editor. | Souied, Eric H., editor. | Querques,
    Giuseppe, editor.
Title: OCT angiography in retinal and macular diseases / volume editors,
    Francesco Bandello, Eric H. Souied, Giuseppe Querques.
Other titles: Optical coherence tomography angiography in retinal and macular
    diseases | Developments in ophthalmology ; v. 56. 0250-3751
Description: Basel ; New York : Karger, 2016. | Series: Developments in
    ophthalmology, ISSN 0250-3751 ; vol. 56 | Includes bibliographical
    references and index.
Identifiers: LCCN 2016002158| ISBN 9783318058291 (hard cover : alk. paper) |
    ISBN 9783318058307 (electronic version)
Subjects: | MESH: Tomography, Optical Coherence | Retinal
    Diseases--radiography | Angiography
Classification: LCC RE79.I42 | NLM WW 270 | DDC 616.07/545--dc23 LC record available at
http://lccn.loc.gov/2016002158

Bibliographic Indices. This publication is listed in bibliographic services, including Current Contents® and Index Medicus.

© Copyright 2016 by S. Karger AG, P.O. Box, CH-4009 Basel (Switzerland)
www.karger.com
Printed in Germany on acid-free and non-aging paper (ISO 9706) by Kraft Druck, Ettlingen
ISSN 0250–3751
e-ISSN 1662–2790
ISBN 978–3–318–05829–1
e-ISBN 978–3–318–05830–7

Contents

V

List of Contributors

Francesco Bandello
Department of Ophthalmology
University Vita Salute
San Raffaele Scientific Institute
Via Olgettina, 60
IT–20132 Milan (Italy)
E-Mail bandello.francesco@hsr.it

Maurizio Battaglia Parodi
Department of Ophthalmology
University Vita Salute
San Raffaele Scientific Institute
Via Olgettina, 60
IT–20132 Milan (Italy)
E-Mail battagliaparodi.maurizio@hsr.it

Caroline R. Baumal
University School of Medicine
New England Eye Center
800 Washington Street, Box 450
Boston, MA 02111 (USA)
E-Mail cbaumal@gmail.com

Susmito Biswas
Manchester Vision Regeneration (MVR) Lab
Research Office, Purple Zone, MRI
Central Manchester University Hospitals NHS
Foundation Trust
Oxford Road
Manchester M13 9WL (UK)
E-Mail Susmito.Biswas@cmft.nhs.uk

Adriano Carnevali
Department of Ophthalmology
University Vita Salute
San Raffaele Scientific Institute
Via Olgettina, 60
IT–20132 Milan (Italy)
E-Mail adrianocarnevali@live.it

Katarzyna Chwiejczak
Manchester Vision Regeneration (MVR) Lab
Research Office, Purple Zone, MRI
Central Manchester University Hospitals NHS
Foundation Trust
Oxford Road
Manchester M13 9WL (UK)
E-Mail Katarzyna.Chwiejczak@cmft.nhs.uk

Salomon Yves Cohen
Department of Ophthalmology
Centre Hospitalier Intercommunal de Créteil
Universite Paris Est Créteil
40 Avenue de Verdun
FR–94000 Créteil (France)
E-Mail sycsyc75@gmail.com

Tim Cole
Topcon House, Kenner Side
Bone Lane
Newbury Berkshire RG14 5PX (UK)
E-Mail tim.cole@topcon.co.uk

Eleonora Corbelli
Department of Ophthalmology
University Vita Salute
San Raffaele Scientific Institute
Via Olgettina, 60
IT–20132 Milan (Italy)
E-Mail corbelli.eleonora@hsr.it

Federico Corvi
Department of Ophthalmology
University Vita Salute
San Raffaele Scientific Institute
Via Olgettina, 60
IT–20132 Milan (Italy)
E-Mail federico.corvi@yahoo.ii

Florence Coscas
Centre Hospitalier Intercommunal de Créteil
40 Avenue de Verdun
FR–94000 Créteil (France)
E-Mail coscas.f@gmail.com

Gabriel Coscas
Centre Hospitalier Intercommunal de Créteil
40 Avenue de Verdun
FR–94000 Créteil (France)
E-Mail gabriel.coscas@gmail.com

Mary K. Durbin
Advanced Development
Carl Zeiss Meditec, Inc.
Dublin, CA 94568 (USA)
E-Mail mary.durbin@zeiss.com

Yvonne D'Souza
Manchester Vision Regeneration (MVR) Lab
Research Office, Purple Zone, MRI
Central Manchester University Hospitals NHS
Foundation Trust
Oxford Road
Manchester M13 9WL (UK)
E-Mail Yvonne.D'Souza@cmft.nhs.uk

Ala El Ameen
Department of Ophthalmology
Centre Hospitalier Intercommunal de Créteil
Universite Paris Est Créteil
40 Avenue de Verdun
FR–94000 Créteil (France)
E-Mail ala-elameen@hotmail.fr

James G. Fujimoto
Department of Electrical Engineering and
Computer Science, Research Laboratory of Electronics
Massachusetts Institute of Technology
77 Massachusetts Avenue, Room 36-361
Cambridge, MA 02139 (USA)
E-Mail jgfuji@mit.edu

Marco Gagliardi
Department of Ophthalmology
University Vita Salute
San Raffaele Scientific Institute
Via Olgettina, 60
IT–20132 Milan (Italy)
E-Mail marco.gagliardi.md@gmail.com

Simon S. Gao
Casey Eye Institute
Oregon Health & Science University
Portland, OR 97239 (USA)
E-Mail gasi@ohsu.edu

Giovanni Gregori
Bascom Palmer Eye Institute
900 NW 17th street
Miami, FL 33136 (USA)
E-Mail GGregori@med.miami.edu

David Huang
Casey Eye Institute
Oregon Health & Science University
Portland, OR 97239 (USA)
E-Mail davidhuang@alum.mit.edu

Nicholas A. Iafe
Stein Eye Institute
David Geffen School of Medicine at UCLA
100 Stein Plaza
Los Angeles, CA 90095 (USA)
E-Mail Niafe@mednet.ucla.edu

Ugo Introini
Department of Ophthalmology
University Vita Salute
San Raffaele Scientific Institute
Via Olgettina, 60
IT–20132 Milan (Italy)
E-Mail introini.ugo@hsr.it

Assad Jalil
Manchester Vision Regeneration (MVR) Lab
Research Office, Purple Zone, MRI
Central Manchester University Hospitals NHS
Foundation Trust
Oxford Road
Manchester M13 9WL (UK)
E-Mail Assad.Jalil@cmft.nhs.uk

Yali Jia
Casey Eye Institute
Oregon Health & Science University
Portland, OR 97239 (USA)
E-Mail jiaya@ohsu.edu

Karen B. Schaal
Bascom Palmer Eye Institute
900 NW 17th street
Miami, FL 33136 (USA)
E-Mail k.schaal@med.miami.edu

Rosangela Lattanzio
Department of Ophthalmology
University Vita Salute, San Raffaele Scientific Institute
Via Olgettina, 60
IT–20132 Milan (Italy)
E-Mail lattanzio.rosangela@hsr.it

Michelle C. Liang
New England Eye Center
Tufts Medical Center
800 Washington Street, Box 450
Boston, MA 02111 (USA)
E-Mail mliang@tuftsmedicalcenter.org

Bruno Lumbroso
Centro Italiano Macula
Via Brofferio 7
IT–00195 Rome (Italy)
E-Mail bruno.lumbroso@gmail.com

Marco Lupidi
Department of Biochemical and Surgical Sciences
Section of Ophthalmology, University of Perugia
S.Maria Della Misericordia Hospital
S.Andrea delle Fratte
IT–06132 Perugia (Italy)
E-Mail dr.marco.lupidi@gmail.com

Alexandra Miere
Department of Ophthalmology
Centre Hospitalier Intercommunal de Créteil
Universite Paris Est Créteil
40 Avenue de Verdun
FR–94000 Créteil (France)
E-Mail alexandramiere@gmail.com

Andrew Miller
Bascom Palmer Eye Institute
900 NW 17th street
Miami, FL 33136 (USA)
E-Mail axm1835@med.miami.edu

Eric M. Moult
Department of Electrical Engineering and
Computer Science, Research Laboratory of Electronics
Massachusetts Institute of Technology
77 Massachusetts Avenue
Room 36-361
Cambridge, MA 02139 (USA)
E-Mail ericmoult@gmail.com

Julia Nemiroff
Stein Eye Institute
David Geffen School of Medicine at University of
California Los Angeles
Los Angeles, CA 90095 (USA)
E-Mail jnemiroff@gmail.com

Eduardo A. Novais
New England Eye Center, Tufts Medical Center
800 Washington Street, Box 450
Boston, MA 02111 (USA)
E-Mail eduardo@novais.md

Alessandro Papayannis
Manchester Vision Regeneration (MVR) Lab
Research Office, Purple Zone, MRI
Central Manchester University Hospitals NHS
Foundation Trust
Oxford Road
Manchester M13 9WL (UK)
E-Mail Alessandro.Papayannis@cmft.nhs.uk

Nopasak Phasukkijwatana
Stein Eye Institute
David Geffen School of Medicine at UCLA
100 Stein Plaza
Los Angeles, CA 90095 (USA)
E-Mail nopasak.sioph@gmail.com

Luisa Pierro
Department of Ophthalmology
University Vita Salute
San Raffaele Scientific Institute
Via Olgettina, 60
IT–20132 Milan (Italy)
E-Mail pierro.luisa@hsr.it

Lea Querques
Department of Ophthalmology
University Vita Salute
San Raffaele Scientific Institute
Via Olgettina, 60
IT–20132 Milan (Italy)
E-Mail querques.lea@hsr.it

Giuseppe Querques
Head – Medical Retina & Imaging Unit
Department of Ophthalmology
University Vita Salute
San Raffaele Scientific Institute
Via Olgettina, 60
IT–20132 Milan (Italy)
E-Mail querques.giuseppe@hsr.it

Alessandro Rabiolo
Department of Ophthalmology
University Vita Salute
San Raffaele Scientific Institute
Via Olgettina, 60
IT–20132 Milan (Italy)
E-Mail rabiolo.alessandro@hsr.it

Marco Rispoli
Centro Italiano Macula
Via Brofferio 7
IT–00195 Rome (Italy)
E-Mail rispolimarco@gmail.com

Gillian Robbins
Bascom Palmer Eye Institute
900 NW 17th street
Miami, FL 33136 (USA)
E-Mail gxr418@med.miami.edu

Luiz Roisman
Bascom Palmer Eye Institute
900 NW 17th street
Miami, FL 33136 (USA)
E-Mail luizroi@yahoo.com.br

Philip J. Rosenfeld
Bascom Palmer Eye Institute
900 NW 17th street
Miami, FL 33136 (USA)
E-Mail prosenfeld@miami.edu

David Sarraf
Stein Eye Institute
David Geffen School of Medicine at UCLA
100 Stein Plaza
Los Angeles, CA 90095 (USA)
E-Mail dsarraf@ucla.edu

Maria Cristina Savastano
Centro Italiano Macula
Via Angelo Brofferio 7
IT–00195 Rome (Italy)
E-Mail crisav8@virgilio.it

Oudy Semoun
Department of Ophthalmology
Centre Hospitalier Intercommunal de Créteil
Universite Paris Est Créteil
40 Avenue de Verdun
FR–94000 Créteil (France)
E-Mail oudysemoun@gmail.com

Eric H. Souied
Department of Ophthalmology
Centre Hospitalier Intercommunal de Créteil
Universite Paris Est Créteil
40 Avenue de Verdun
FR–94000 Créteil (France)
E-Mail eric.souied@chicreteil.fr

Mayer Srour
Department of Ophthalmology
Centre Hospitalier Intercommunal de Créteil
Universite Paris Est Créteil
40 Avenue de Verdun
FR–94000 Créteil (France)
E-Mail srour.mayer@gmail.com

Paulo E. Stanga
Manchester Vision Regeneration (MVR) Lab
Research Office, Purple Zone, MRI
Central Manchester University Hospitals NHS
Foundation Trust
Oxford Road
Manchester M13 9WL (UK)
E-Mail Paulo.Stanga@cmft.nhs.uk

Francesco Stringa
Manchester Vision Regeneration (MVR) Lab
Research Office, Purple Zone, MRI
Central Manchester University Hospitals NHS
Foundation Trust
Oxford Road
Manchester M13 9WL (UK)
E-Mail mvr.lab@cmft.nhs.uk

Ou Tan
Casey Eye Institute
Oregon Health & Science University
Portland, OR 97239 (USA)
E-Mail tano@ohsu.edu

Emmanouil Tsamis
Manchester Vision Regeneration (MVR) Lab
Research Office, Purple Zone, MRI
Central Manchester University Hospitals NHS
Foundation Trust
Oxford Road
Manchester M13 9WL (UK)
E-Mail emmanouil.tsamis@manchester.ac.uk

Nadia K. Waheed
New England Eye Center at Tufts Medical Center
260 Tremont Street
Boston, MA 02116 (USA)
E-Mail nadiakwaheed@gmail.com

Andre J. Witkin
New England Eye Center
Tufts Medical Center
800 Washington Street, Box 450
Boston, MA 02111 (USA)
E-Mail awitkin@tuftsmedicalcenter.org

Fang Zheng
Bascom Palmer Eye Institute
900 NW 17th street
Miami, FL 33136 (USA)
E-Mail fxz99@miami.edu

Preface

The feeling that we have, as retina specialists, is that we are going to live through a revolutionary change: the introduction of optical coherence tomography angiography as a routine exam in clinical practice is already modifying the approach to patients, giving us the opportunity to investigate retinal and choroidal circulation in a noninvasive way.

For sure, we all are still trying to interpret the information, and many of the images that we get still need a great effort to be understood. However, it is undoubtable that the way that we look at our patients is going to change thanks to the introduction of this new methodology.

In this book, many of the major experts (and friends) who joined us as speakers at the 2nd San Raffaele OCT Forum agreed to share their experiences and contributed the latest images and ideas.

We sincerely hope that our efforts will be useful to all of you who are starting to be involved in this new era, and in few years, we are sure, we all will use new diagnostic paradigms with a significant improvement of quality of care for our patients.

We are grateful to the companies that helped in the realization of this initiative (Heidelberg, Optovue, Topcon, Zeiss). They will be our companions during the next years, and we hope that they will help us to obtain new, better-performing devices.

We would also like to thank Karger, which made this book possible in only a few months by working very hard, and finally, we express our gratitude to all doctors, technicians and nurses who share their enthusiasm and efforts with us daily.

This book is dedicated to our mentors Prof. Rosario Brancato and Prof. Gabriel Coscas. Their passion for the retina initiated us into our professional lives.

Lastly, we thank our patients. We work for them, but without them, nothing would be possible.

Enjoy reading,

Francesco Bandello, Milan
Eric H. Souied, Créteil
Giuseppe Querques, Milan

Bandello F, Souied EH, Querques G (eds): OCT Angiography in Retinal and Macular Diseases.
Dev Ophthalmol. Basel, Karger, 2016, vol 56, pp 1–5 (DOI: 10.1159/000442768)

Heidelberg Spectralis Optical Coherence Tomography Angiography: Technical Aspects

Gabriel Coscas[a, b] · Marco Lupidi[a, c] · Florence Coscas[a, b]

[a]Centre de l'Odéon, Paris, and [b]Department of Ophthalmology, Centre Hospitalier Intercommunal de Créteil, Université Paris Est, Créteil, France; [c]Department of Biomedical and Surgical Sciences, Section of Ophthalmology, University of Perugia, S. Maria della Misericordia Hospital, Perugia, Italy

Abstract

Optical coherence tomography angiography (OCT-A) is a promising new method for visualizing the retinal vasculature and choroidal vascular layers in the macular area and provides depth-resolved functional information on blood flow in these vessels. OCT-A is based on the concept that in a static eye the *only* moving structure in the fundus of the eye is blood flowing through the vessels. Contrast is generated based on the difference between moving cells in the vasculature and the static surrounding tissue. Artifacts can arise due to scan positioning errors caused by normal ocular microsaccades. In order to avoid artifacts, a sequence of OCT B-scans in the exact same retinal location must be taken to detect flow. Active eye-tracking (TruTrack™) using the simultaneous acquisition of fundus and optical coherence tomography (OCT) images presents a very reliable method of acquiring OCT volume scans *without motion artifacts* and helps significantly improve signal-to-noise ratio. This system also allows the use of a full spectrum amplitude decorrelation algorithm that produces clear differentiation between blood flow and static tissue without sacrificing the axial resolution of OCT images. Accuracy in layer segmentation, which requires high-resolution OCT B-scans, is crucial for producing reliable OCT-A images. This can be achieved through automated or manual layer segmentation. During OCT scan acquisition, the effect of axial motion (e.g. a patient moving towards the camera) is compensated for by geometric alignment of successive B-scans before analyzing temporal changes.

© 2016 S. Karger AG, Basel

Introduction

Optical coherence tomography angiography (OCT-A) is a promising new method for visualizing the retinal vasculature and choroidal vascular layers in the macular area.

A key advantage of OCT-A over traditional fluorescein angiography (FA) is that it provides depth-resolved functional information of blood flow in vessels.

In comparison, FA provides only a bi-dimensional image that superimposes all perfused layers of retinal and choroidal blood vessels.

OCT-A images often appear similar to FA images when viewed as C-scans, but they provide additional information.

For correct interpretation of the images, it is important to understand the differences between the two modalities.

Spectralis OCT2 Device

The Spectralis OCT2 device (Spectralis, Heidelberg Engineering, Heidelberg, Germany) is a prototype device that is able to acquire 85,000 A-scans per second, with an axial resolution of 7 μm, a lateral resolution of 14 μm, and a bandwidth of 50 nm. An amplitude decorrelation algorithm developed by Heidelberg Engineering (Heidelberg, Germany) is applied to a volume scan on a $15 \times 5°$ or $15 \times 10°$ area (4.3×1.5 mm or 4.3×2.9 mm), which is composed of a variable number of B-scans (ranging from 131 to 261, respectively) at a distance of 11 μm each (this value is very near the limit of eyesight resolution).

In its automated real-time mode, the prototype device allows a variable number of frames per scan in order to average an image, increase the quality of each single B-scan and improve the signal-to-noise ratio.

A B-scan in OCT-A mode is generated by computing the decorrelation in between successive standard B-scans that are sequentially acquired at the same location.

The decorrelation between each acquired B-scan and a second scan taken in the same location is assessed in order to obtain an optical coherence tomography (OCT) B-scan angiogram. Since OCT-A is simultaneously achieved with the corresponding standard OCT B-scan, both retinal/choroidal functional aspects and morphological aspects are visualized.

Genesis of Optical Coherence Tomography Angiograms

OCT-A is based on the concept that in a static eye the *only* moving structure in the fundus of the eye is blood flowing through its vessels.

Contrast is generated based on the difference between moving cells in the vasculature and the static surrounding tissue.

Different contributing factors need to be considered. When performing OCT scans of the retina, the main sources of motion are bulk motion and motion caused by circulating blood.

Bulk motion refers to any movement of tissue with respect to an OCT device; this includes head movements and eye movements. If bulk motions are sufficiently compensated, then blood circulation is the predominant source of temporal changes between OCT scans.

Motion can also be caused by *circulating blood.* OCT can therefore be used to visualize blood flow based on the detection of temporal changes within a sequence of scans.

Artifacts can arise due to scan positioning errors caused by normal ocular microsaccades.

They commonly occur once every 300 ms (while a typical acquisition time for OCT volume scanning, with a reasonable resolution and field of view, takes at least 2–3 s to acquire).

In order to avoid the creation of artifacts, a sequence of OCT B-scans must be taken at the exact same retinal location to detect flow (fig. 1).

Role of Eye-Tracking System

The use of an active eye-tracking system (TruTrack™, Heidelberg Engineering, Heidelberg, Germany) enables the acquisition of very reliable OCT volume scans *without motion artifacts.*

The eye-tracking method is based on the simultaneous acquisition of fundus and OCT images. The method makes it possible to perform a

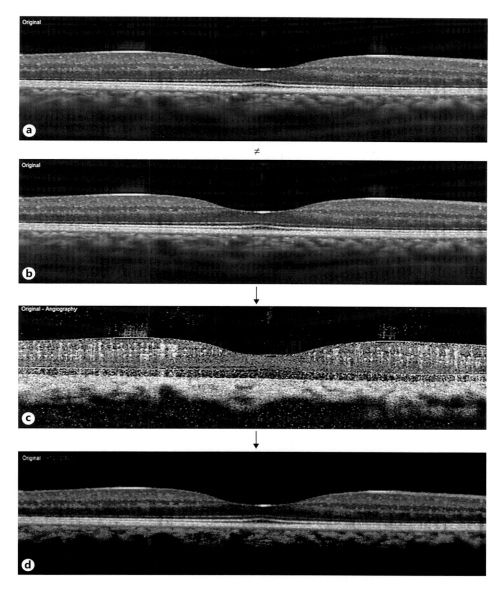

Fig. 1. Principles of optical coherence tomography angiography (OCT-A). **a** Acquired B-scan. **b** A second B-scan, taken in the exact same retinal location. **c** OCT B-scan angiogram. **d** OCT B-scan in an overlapped mode. The difference between an acquired B-scan (**a**) and a second one taken in the exact same retinal location (**b**) is computed in order to obtain a decorrelation signal. This decorrelation signal, which is mainly due to blood cells flowing through vessels, is used to create an OCT B-scan angiogram (**c**). Morphological (conventional OCT) and functional (OCT-A) information may be simultaneously shown in an overlapped mode (**d**).

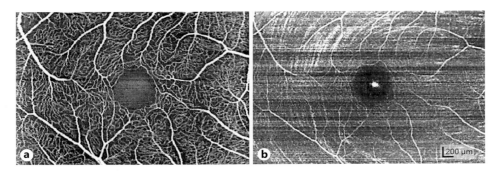

Fig. 2. Comparison between OCT-A and conventional 'en face' OCT C-scans. C-scan in OCT-A mode. Conventional 'en face' C-scan. A C-scan in OCT-A mode (**a**) allows clear 'en face' visualization of different vascular layers, which are well defined and can be distinguished from avascular areas. On the contrary, a conventional C-scan (**b**) shows only the larger trunks of retinal vessels, which appear as hyperreflective structures. The whole image is also not fully interpretable due to the reflectivity of the retinal nerve fiber layer, which focally masks the image of the deeper structures.

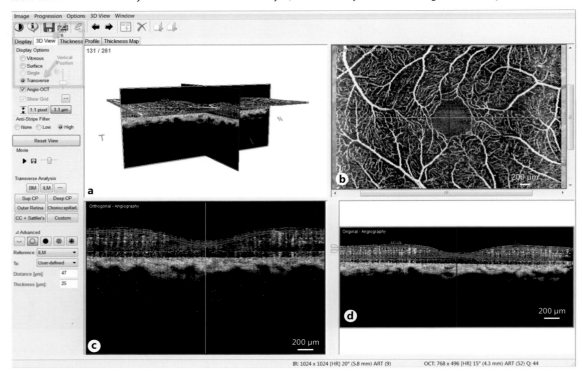

Fig. 3. Spectralis OCT-A screen visualization. Aspect of Spectralis OCT-A in Heyex Software (Heyex Software Version 1.9.201.0, Heidelberg Engineering, Heidelberg, Germany). The shown 4-picture view can be obtained by selecting '3D View' in the upper bar and simultaneously selecting 'Transverse' in the display options (yellow box and arrows). Combined visualization of three other planes (**b–d**) is useful for analyzing the spatial relationship between them. **b** 'En face' visualization of an OCT-A scan showing the superficial capillary plexus of a healthy subject. Two lines, one horizontal (green) and one vertical (blue), identify the exact positions of the two B-scans shown in (**c**) and (**d**). **c** Orthogonal B-scan in angio-mode (corresponding to blue line in fig. (**b**)) is useful for evaluating segmentation algorithm quality (red lines). **d** Original B-scan in angio-mode (corresponding to green line in fig. (**b**)) shows one single B-scan extracted from a volume scan of a 15 × 10° region centered in the macular area.

continuous real-time quality check of OCT data during an exam. This process ensures that only accurate OCT images are stored.

Therefore, as part of a clinical routine, a physician (and/or technician or photographer) will not need to schedule a reexamination of a patient if eye movement or blinking occurred during an acquisition. The TruTrack™ system significantly helps improve the signal-to-noise ratio.

Full-Spectrum Amplitude Decorrelation Algorithm

Employing an eye-tracking system also allows the use of a full-spectrum amplitude decorrelation algorithm. This guarantees clear differentiation between blood flow and static tissue without sacrificing axial resolution (i.e. depth resolution) in OCT images. In this way, very thin layers of the vascular network become distinguishable in C-scan sections.

The effect of *axial motion* (e.g. a patient moving towards the camera) must be compensated for as well. Our approach is to geometrically align successive B-scans before performing an analysis of temporal changes. This is done during OCT scan acquisition. In this case, blood flow can be identified even when strong bulk motion occurs during acquisition.

C-Scan ('en face') Visualization in Optical Coherence Tomography Angiography

C-scan ('en face') visualization in OCT-A is automatically derived from OCT B-scan angiograms. The use of automated real-time mode, which facilitates effective discrimination between image 'noise' and true signals from real tissue structures, is associated with the limited distance in between two consecutive B-scans (11 µm) and allows the best high-resolution C-scan angiogram to be obtained (fig. 2).

Overall, OCT-A with active eye-tracking and proper B-scan alignment yields desirable definition and high geometrical accuracy. To achieve high-resolution OCT-A scans, dense OCT volume scans must be acquired, and each single B-scan of a volume protocol must be of consistent high quality (fig. 3).

Prof. Gabriel Coscas
Centre Hospitalier Intercommunal de Créteil
40 Avenue de Verdun
FR–94000 Créteil (France)
E-Mail gabriel.coscas@gmail.com

Bandello F, Souied EH, Querques G (eds): OCT Angiography in Retinal and Macular Diseases.
Dev Ophthalmol. Basel, Karger, 2016, vol 56, pp 6–12 (DOI: 10.1159/000442770)

Optical Coherence Tomography Angiography Using the Optovue Device

David Huang[a] · Yali Jia[a] · Simon S. Gao[a] · Bruno Lumbroso[b] · Marco Rispoli[b]

[a]Casey Eye Institute, Oregon Health and Science University, Portland, Oreg., USA; [b]Centro Italiano Macula, Rome, Italy

Abstract

Optovue AngioVue system technology for optical coherence tomography (OCT) angiography is based on the AngioVue Imaging System (Optovue, Inc., Freemont, CA), using split-spectrum amplitude-decorrelation angiography (SSADA) algorithm. This algorithm was developed to minimize scanning time. It detects motion in blood vessel lumen by measuring the variation in reflected OCT signal amplitude between consecutive cross-sectional scans. The novelty of SSADA lies in how the OCT signal is processed to enhance flow detection and reject axial bulk motion noise. Specifically, the algorithm splits the OCT image into different spectral bands, thus increasing the number of usable image frames. Each new frame has a lower axial resolution that is less susceptible to axial eye motion caused by blood pulsation. Optovue AngioVue system technology allows quantitative analysis. It provides numerical data about flow area and non-flow area. It can also generate a flow density map. These metrics may serve as biomarkers in diagnosis and for tracking disease progression or treatment response. Flow area: the software will calculate the drawn area and vessel area in mm². It allows for comparison of all measurements for a given participant. Non-flow area: the software shows the non-perfused areas by mouse click selection. Ischemic areas will be shown in yellow. These areas may be saved and matched with others in the study. Flow density tool is able to measure the percentage of vascular areas on en face angiograms. This analysis is based on an ETDRS grid centered on the macula as with the thickness map. This tool works both on inner and outer vascular plexus.

© 2016 S. Karger AG, Basel

The Optovue AngioVue system is used for optical coherence tomography angiography (OCT-A), employing technology based on the AngioVue imaging system (Optovue, Inc., Freemont, CA). This instrument has an A-scan rate of 70,000 scans per second using a light source centered on 840 nm and a bandwidth of 50 nm. Each OCT-A volume contains 304 × 304 A-scans with two consecutive B-scans captured at each fixed position before proceeding to the next sampling location.

Split-spectrum amplitude-decorrelation angiography (SSADA) is used to extract the OCT-A information. Each OCT-A volume is acquired in 3 seconds, and two orthogonal OCT-A volumes are acquired for orthogonal registration using motion correction technology [1, 2] to minimize motion artifacts arising from microsaccades and fixation changes. Angiography information is displayed as the maximum of the decorrelation values when viewed perpendicularly through the thickness being evaluated.

The Avanti Widefield optical coherence tomography (OCT) system is a spectral domain OCT system that is the platform for Optovue's OCT-A technology. When the OCT-A software is installed, it becomes an AngioVue system.

Optical Coherence Tomography Angiography

Initially, Doppler OCT-A methods were investigated for the visualization and measurement of blood flow [3–8]. Because Doppler OCT is sensitive only to motion parallel to an OCT probe beam, it is limited in its ability to image retinal and choroidal circulation, which are predominantly perpendicular to the OCT beam. An alternative approach is speckle-based OCT-A. This approach has advantages over Doppler-based techniques because it uses variations in speckle patterns over time to detect both transverse and axial flow with similar sensitivities. Amplitude-based [9–11], phase-based [12], or combined amplitude+phase [13] variance methods have been described.

Split-Spectrum Amplitude-Decorrelation Angiography

The SSADA algorithm was developed to minimize scanning time. It detects motion in blood vessel lumen by measuring variations in reflected OCT signal amplitude between consecutive cross-sectional scans. Decorrelation is a mathematical function that quantifies variation without being affected by the average signal strength, as long as the signal is strong enough to predominate over optical and electronic noise. The novelty of SSADA lies in how the OCT signal is processed to enhance flow detection and reject axial bulk motion noise. Specifically, the algorithm splits an OCT image into different spectral bands, thus increasing the number of usable image frames. Each new frame has a lower axial resolution that is less susceptible to axial eye motion caused by retrobulbar pulsation. This lower resolution also translates to a wider coherence gate over which the reflected signal from a moving particle, such as a blood cell, can interfere with adjacent structures, thereby increasing speckle contrast. In addition, each spectral band contains a different speckle pattern and independent information on flow. When amplitude-decorrelation images from multiple spectral bands are combined, the flow signal is increased. Compared to the full-spectrum amplitude method, SSADA using four-fold spectral splits can improve the signal-to-noise ratio by a factor of two, which is equivalent to reducing the scan time by a factor of four [14]. More recent SSADA implementations use an eleven-fold split to further enhance the signal-to-noise ratio of flow detection [15]. As shown by an example from *en face* angiograms of the macular retinal circulation collected using a commercial 70 kHz, 840-nm wavelength spectral OCT device (fig. 1), SSADA provides a clean and continuous microvascular network and less noise just inside the foveal avascular zone.

As OCT-A generates 3D data, segmentation and *en face* presentation of flow information can aid in reducing data complexity and serve to reproduce the more traditional view of dye-based angiography. As seen in fig. 1, the retinal angiogram (fig. 1b–d) represents the decorrelation or flow information between the internal limiting membrane and the outer plexiform layer. Segmentation performed on cross-sectional, struc-

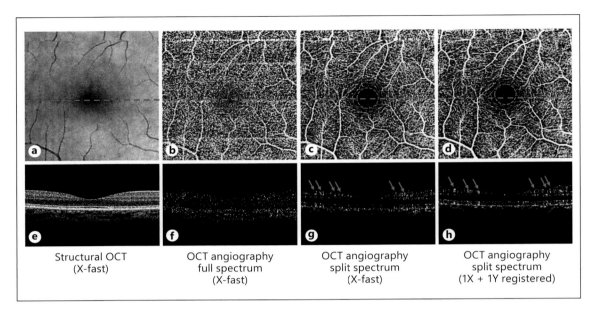

| Structural OCT (X-fast) | OCT angiography full spectrum (X-fast) | OCT angiography split spectrum (X-fast) | OCT angiography split spectrum (1X + 1Y registered) |

Fig. 1. Comparison of structural optical coherence tomography (OCT) (**a**, **e**) and amplitude-decorrelation angiograms of the macula (3 × 3 mm area) using full-spectrum (**b**, **f**), split-spectrum (**c**, **g**), and split-spectrum averaged angiograms from one X-fast and one F-fast scans after 3D registration (**d**, **h**). *En face* maximum decorrelation projections of retinal circulation showed less noise inside the foveal avascular zone (within the green dotted circles) and more continuous perifoveal vascular networks using the split-spectrum amplitude-decorrelation angiography algorithm (**c**) compared to the standard full-spectrum algorithm (**b**). Cross-sectional angiograms (scanned across the red dashed lines in **b** and **c**) showed more clearly delineated retinal vessels (red arrows in **g**) and less noise using the split-spectrum amplitude-decorrelation angiography algorithm (**g**) compared to the standard (**f**). There are saccadic motion artifacts that appear as artifactual horizontal lines in (**b**, **c**). These and other motion artifacts are removed using a 3D registration algorithm that registers horizontal-priority (X-fast) and a vertical-priority (Y-fast) raster scans to remove motion error. The algorithm then merges the X-fast and Y-fast scans to produce a merged 3D OCT angiogram[2] that shows a continuous artifact-free microvascular network, as shown in (**d**). The registration and averaging of two orthogonal scans also removed motion blur and further improved signal-to-noise ratio, allowing the visualization of a greater number of distinct small retinal vessels (microvascular network in **d**, red arrows in **h**). Reproduced with permission from 'Manuale Pratico di Angiografia OCT'; Fabiano Publisher 2015.

tural OCT images (fig. 1e) can be directly applied to the OCT-A images (fig. 1f and g). The *en face* angiograms were generated by projecting the maximum decorrelation or flow value for each transverse position within the segmented depth range, representing the fastest flowing vessel lumen in the segmented tissue layers. In healthy eyes, the retinal angiogram shows a vascular network around the foveal avascular zone. The layers of the retina and choroid can be more finely separated (fig. 2) to provide additional information to define diagnostic parameters of vascular defects.

Relationship between Decorrelation and Velocity

To determine how the decorrelation or flow signal produced by the SSADA algorithm relates to flow velocity, phantom experiments were performed [16]. The study showed that SSADA is sensitive to both axial and transverse flow, with a slightly higher sensitivity for the axial component. For clinical retinal imaging where the OCT beam is approximately perpendicular to the vasculature, for all practical purposes, the

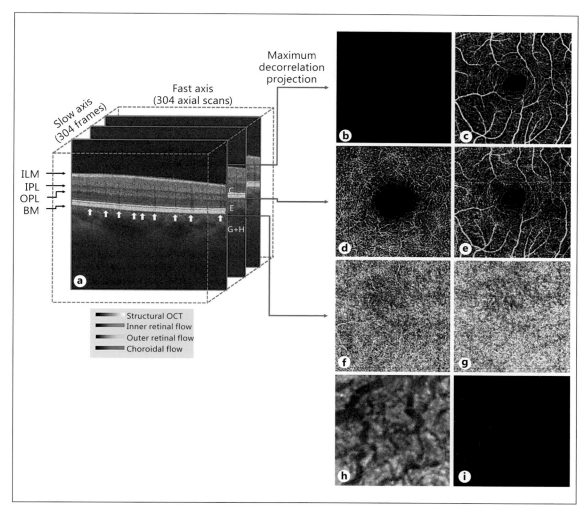

Fig. 2. Segmentation and processing of an OCT angiogram of a normal macula. **a** The 3D OCT angiogram comprises 304 frames of averaged decorrelation cross-sections stretched along the slow scan axis. **a** The cross-sectional angiogram shows that flow in the inner retinal vessels (purple) are projected onto bright photoreceptor and retinal pigment epithelium layers (indicated by white arrows). Image processing software separates the vitreous, inner retinal layers, outer retinal layer, and choroidal layers along the inner limiting membrane, outer boundary of the inner plexiform layer, outer boundary of the outer plexiform layer, and Bruch's membrane (dotted green lines). Six segmented flow volumes are separately projected. The projection algorithm finds the maximum decorrelation value for each transverse position within the segmented depth range, representing the fastest flowing vessel lumen in the segmented tissue layers. **b** The vitreous angiogram shows the absence of vascular flow. **c** The superficial inner retinal angiogram shows normal retinal circulation with a small foveal avascular zone of approximately 0.6 mm in diameter. **d** The deep inner retina angiogram shows the deep retinal plexus, which is a network of fine vessels. **e** The outer retina slab shows flow projection artifacts cast by flowing blood in the inner retinal vessels onto the retinal pigment epithelium. **f** A choriocapillaris angiogram. **g** A deeper choroid angiogram. **h** A deeper choroid *en face* structural OCT. **i** An outer retinal angiogram after removal of the projection artifact using a post-processing algorithm. Reproduced with permission from 'Manuale Pratico di Angiografia OCT'; Fabiano Publisher 2015.

SSADA signal can be considered to be independent of the small variation in beam incidence angle. In addition, it was found that decorrelation was linearly related to velocity over a limited range. A higher decorrelation value thus implies higher velocity flow. This range is dependent on the time scale of the SSADA measurement. With a 70 kHz spectral OCT system and 200+ A-scans per cross-sectional B-scan, SSADA should be sensitive to even the slowest flow at the capillary level, where flow speeds have been estimated at between 0.4 and 3 mm/s [17, 18]. In larger vessels with higher velocities, the SSADA signal reaches a maximum value (saturates).

Limitations of Optical Coherence Tomography Angiography

OCT-A has several limitations. First, shadowgraphic flow projection artifacts make the interpretation of *en face* angiograms of deeper vascular beds more difficult. These artifacts are a result of fluctuating shadows cast by flowing blood in a superficial vascular layer that cause variations in OCT signal in deeper, highly reflective layers. The flow projection artifact from the retinal circulation can be seen clearly on the bright retinal pigment epithelium. This artifact can be removed by software processing. The projection from the retinal circulation is relatively sparse and can be removed from deeper layers fairly effectively. However, the choriocapillaris is nearly confluent, and its projection and shadow effects are difficult to remove from deeper choroidal layers. A second limitation is the fading of OCT and flow signal in large vessels due to the interferometric fringe washout effect associated with very fast blood flow, especially the axial flow component [19]. This means that central retinal vessels in the disc and large vessels in the deep choroid cannot be visualized using SSADA. Third, the scan area of OCT-A is relatively small

(3 × 3 to 6 × 6 mm). Larger-area angiograms of high quality can be achieved, but require higher speed OCT systems that are not yet commercially available [20]. Lastly, because OCT-A best resolves pathology when viewed as *en face* angiograms of anatomic layers, practical clinical applications require accurate segmentation software. Post-processing software is also needed to reduce motion and projection artifacts. The need for these sophisticated algorithms means that OCT-A still has much room to improve in the foreseeable future.

Comparing Swept-Source and Spectral Optical Coherence Tomography

The SSADA algorithm was initially implemented on a custom-built 100 kHz, 1,050-nm wavelength swept-source OCT system. To generate high-quality angiograms (fig. 3a), 8 consecutive cross-sectional scans at each position were necessary. A scan pattern of 200 cross-sectional scan positions, each with 200 axial scans, was used. The overall angiographic scan pattern had 200 × 200 transverse points. A total of 200 × 200 × 8 axial scans were acquired in 3.5 seconds.

The commercial implementation of SSADA uses a 70 kHz, 840-nm wavelength spectral OCT system. Although this system acquires fewer axial scans per second, high-quality angiograms with more transverse points (304 × 304, fig. 3b) are produced in less time (3 seconds). The higher performance is due to the lower decorrelation noise on the spectral OCT system, which requires only 2 consecutive cross-sectional scans at one position to compute a reliable decorrelation image. The higher transverse scan density, along with the higher transverse resolution associated with the shorter wavelength, means that the Avanti produces retinal angiograms with higher definition and higher resolution than the swept-source OCT prototype that was originally used (fig. 3c and d).

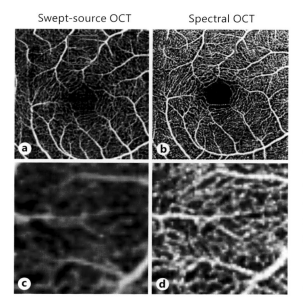

Swept-source OCT   Spectral OCT

Fig. 3. Comparison of 3 × 3 mm macular angiograms from a 100 kHz swept-source OCT system (**a**) and 70 kHz spectral OCT system (**b**). Zoomed-in views shows improved capillary detail from the spectral OCT system (**d**) compared to the swept-source OCT system (**c**). Reproduced with permission from 'Manuale Pratico di Angiografia OCT'; Fabiano Publisher 2015.

Quantitative Analysis

The latest developments for OCT-A relate to methods for quantitative analysis of OCT angiograms [21–25]. Optovue's new quantification tool is called AngioAnalytics, and it provides numerical data about flow area and nonflow area. AngioAnalytics can also generate a flow density map. These metrics may serve as biomarkers in diagnosis and for tracking disease progression or treatment response.

Flow Area

Flow area is useful in cases of choroidal neovascularization and preretinal neovascularization during diabetic retinopathy or vascular vein occlusion. In these pathologies, traditional angiography shows new vessels masked by leakage and staining, while OCT-A allows for direct and clear visualization of the vascular network. In Angio-Analytics, the operator draws the choroidal neovascularization boundary, and the software will then calculate the drawn area and vessel area in mm^2. Furthermore, it allows for comparison of all measurements for a given participant.

Nonflow Area

Nonflow area represents the vascular dropout area. These are regions where there is no detectable flow by SSADA. This tool seems to be useful in all ischemic retinopathies caused by various etiologies. With OCT-A, it is possible to separate the inner and deep vascular plexus. After proper *en face* projection, the software will show the nonperfused areas by mouse click selection. Ischemic areas will be shown in yellow. These areas may be saved and matched with others in the study.

Flow Density Map

This tool is able to measure the percentage of vascular areas on *en face* angiograms. This analysis is based on an Early Treatment Diabetic Retinopathy Study grid centered on the macula, as with the thickness map. This tool works on both the inner and outer vascular plexus.

References

1 Kraus MF, Liu JJ, Schottenhamml J, et al: Quantitative 3D-OCT motion correction with tilt and illumination correction, robust similarity measure and regularization. Biomed Opt Express 2014;5: 2591–2613.

2 Kraus MF, Potsaid B, Mayer MA, et al: Motion correction in optical coherence tomography volumes on a per A-scan basis using orthogonal scan patterns. Biomed Opt Express 2012;3:1182–1199.

3 Wang RK, Jacques SL, Ma Z, et al: Three dimensional optical angiography. Opt Express 2007;15:4083–4097.

4 Grulkowski I, Gorczynska I, Szkulmowski M, et al: Scanning protocols dedicated to smart velocity ranging in Spectral OCT. Opt Express 2009;17:23736–23754.

5 Yu L, Chen Z: Doppler variance imaging for three-dimensional retina and choroid angiography. J Biomed Opt 2010; 15:016029.

6 Makita S, Jaillon F, Yamanari M, et al: Comprehensive in vivo micro-vascular imaging of the human eye by dual-beam-scan Doppler optical coherence angiography. Opt Express 2011;19: 1271–1283.

7 Zotter S, Pircher M, Torzicky T, et al: Visualization of microvasculature by dual-beam phase-resolved Doppler optical coherence tomography. Opt Express 2011;19:1217–1227.

8 Braaf B, Vermeer KA, Vienola KV, de Boer JF: Angiography of the retina and the choroid with phase-resolved OCT using interval-optimized backstitched B-scans. Opt Express 2012;20:20516–20534.

9 Mariampillai A, Standish BA, Moriyama EH, et al: Speckle variance detection of microvasculature using swept-source optical coherence tomography. Opt Lett 2008;33:1530–1532.

10 Motaghiannezam R, Fraser S: Logarithmic intensity and speckle-based motion contrast methods for human retinal vasculature visualization using swept source optical coherence tomography. Biomed Opt Express 2012;3:503–521.

11 Enfield J, Jonathan E, Leahy M: In vivo imaging of the microcirculation of the volar forearm using correlation mapping optical coherence tomography (cmOCT). Biomed Opt Express 2011;2: 1184–1193.

12 Fingler J, Zawadzki RJ, Werner JS, et al: Volumetric microvascular imaging of human retina using optical coherence tomography with a novel motion contrast technique. Opt Express 2009;17: 22190–22200.

13 Liu G, Lin AJ, Tromberg BJ, et al: A comparison of Doppler optical coherence tomography methods. Biomed Opt Express 2012;3:2669–2680.

14 Jia Y, Tan O, Tokayer J, et al: Split-spectrum amplitude-decorrelation angiography with optical coherence tomography. Opt Express 2012;20:4710–4725.

15 Gao SS, Liu G, Huang D, et al: Optimization of the split-spectrum amplitude-decorrelation angiography algorithm on a spectral optical coherence tomography system. Opt Lett 2015;40:2305–2308.

16 Tokayer J, Jia Y, Dhalla AH, et al: Blood flow velocity quantification using split-spectrum amplitude-decorrelation angiography with optical coherence tomography. Biomed Opt Express 2013;4: 1909–1924.

17 Riva CE, Petrig B: Blue field entoptic phenomenon and blood velocity in the retinal capillaries. J Opt Soc Am 1980; 70:1234–1238.

18 Tam J, Tiruveedhula P, Roorda A: Characterization of single-file flow through human retinal parafoveal capillaries using an adaptive optics scanning laser ophthalmoscope. Biomed Opt Express 2011;2:781–793.

19 Hendargo HC, McNabb RP, Dhalla A-H, et al: Doppler velocity detection limitations in spectrometer-based versus swept-source optical coherence tomography. Biomed Opt Express 2011;2: 2175–2188.

20 Blatter C, Klein T, Grajciar B, et al: Ultrahigh-speed non-invasive widefield angiography. J Biomed Opt 2012;17: 0705051–0705053.

21 Jia Y, Bailey ST, Hwang TS, et al: Quantitative optical coherence tomography angiography of vascular abnormalities in the living human eye. Proc Natl Acad Sci U S A 2015;112:E2395–E2402.

22 Jia Y, Bailey ST, Wilson DJ, et al: Quantitative optical coherence tomography angiography of choroidal neovascularization in age-related macular degeneration. Ophthalmology 2014;121:1435–1444.

23 Jia Y, Wei E, Wang X, et al: Optical coherence tomography angiography of optic disc perfusion in glaucoma. Ophthalmology 2014;121:1322–1332.

24 Liu L, Gao SS, Bailey ST, et al: Automated choroidal neovascularization detection algorithm for optical coherence tomography angiography. Biomed Opt Express 2015;6:3564–3576.

25 Agemy SA, Scripsema NK, Shah CM, et al: Retinal vascular perfusion density mapping using optical coherence tomography angiography in normals and diabetic retinopathy patients. Retina 2015;35:2353–2363.

Bruno Lumbroso
Centro Italiano Macula
Via Brofferio 7
IT–00195 Rome (Italy)
E-Mail bruno.lumbroso@gmail.com

Bandello F, Souied EH, Querques G (eds): OCT Angiography in Retinal and Macular Diseases.
Dev Ophthalmol. Basel, Karger, 2016, vol 56, pp 13–17 (DOI: 10.1159/000442771)

Swept-Source Optical Coherence Tomography Angio™ (Topcon Corp, Japan): Technology Review

Paulo E. Stanga[a–c] · Emmanouil Tsamis[a–c] · Alessandro Papayannis[a, b] · Francesco Stringa[a] · Tim Cole[d] · Assad Jalil[a, b]

[a]Manchester Vision Regeneration (MVR) Lab at Manchester Royal Eye Hospital & NIHR/Wellcome Trust Manchester CRF, Manchester, [b]Manchester Royal Eye Hospital, Central Manchester University Hospitals NHS Foundation Trust, Manchester, [c]Institute of Human Development, Faculty of Medical and Human Sciences, University of Manchester, Manchester, and [d]Topcon (GB) Ltd., Newbury, UK

Abstract

Optical coherence tomography (OCT) angiography (OCTA) is a novel, noninvasive, three-dimensional imaging technique that allows for the visualization of intravascular flow in the microvasculature. Swept-source OCT technology utilizes longer-wavelength infrared light than conventional spectral-domain OCT. This enables improved penetration into tissue and imaging through optical opacities and is invisible to the subject. Topcon has recently developed an innovative OCTA algorithm, OCTARA (OCTA Ratio Analysis), which benefits from being paired with swept-source OCT. OCTARA aims to provide improved detection sensitivity of low blood flow and reduced motion artifacts without compromising axial resolution. In this chapter, we describe the implementation of OCTARA with swept-source OCT technology, the technical specifications of acquisition (e.g. the number of scans, area of examination field, etc.) along with the algorithm's function and principles for analysis of B-scan data to achieve angiographic visualization. Examples of OCTA scans performed using the OCTARA algorithm and a comparison of these scans with images obtained using other technologies are also presented.

© 2016 S. Karger AG, Basel

Optical coherence tomography (OCT) angiography (OCTA) is a novel, noninvasive, three-dimensional imaging technique that can be used to visualize intravascular flow at the microcirculation level [1–3]. It is performed within a few seconds without the injection of any dye and without causing any discomfort.

An innovative OCTA algorithm that aims to provide improved detection sensitivity of low blood flow and reduced motion artifacts without compromising axial resolution has recently been developed by Topcon (Topcon Corporation,

Tokyo, Japan). Topcon's OCTA implementation further benefits from being paired with swept-source (SS) OCT technology, given the high 100 kHz A-line rate, 1 μm-wavelength light source, and deep signal penetration through the retina and choroid. SS-OCT utilizes longer-wavelength infrared light than conventional spectral-domain OCT and therefore has improved penetration into tissue, can image through optical opacities and is invisible to the subject. This technology also does not suffer significant signal roll-off compared with spectral-domain OCT, which requires enhanced depth imaging techniques to visualize the choroid.

Using a DRI OCT imaging system, SS-OCT technology can acquire 100,000 A-scans per second in both healthy and diseased eyes. Volumetric OCT scans can be acquired over a 3 × 3 mm field of view in about 4 seconds of total OCT scan time. Each B-scan position is repeatedly scanned 4 times. The examination field can be enlarged to 6 × 6 mm (Triton and Atlantis) or even to 12 × 9 mm (Atlantis prototype only).

IMAGEnet® 6, a web-based ophthalmic data management system, incorporates visualization of angiographic data sets, providing both standard and customizable *en-face* and cross-sectional views of OCTA data in conjunction with corresponding structural data.

OCTA methods are generally based on quantification of motion contrast. In a practical implementation, a single location may be scanned two or more times to obtain ocular B-scan data. A calculation is performed across corresponding pixels in each frame or combination of frames to quantify the degree of motion contrast. This measure is then presumed to correspond to angiographic flow, as blood flow is the primary cause of signal change under normal imaging conditions after bulk motion has been accounted for. Some angiographic methods compute the differences between image frames, whereas others may compute the variance over an arbitrary number of frames.

Various companies have used different calculation methods to analyze OCT intensity information, from the measurement of speckle variance, which was first demonstrated by A. Mariampillai et al. [1], to the measurement of simple decorrelation while simultaneously splitting the spectrum into smaller bands (split-spectrum amplitude-decorrelation angiography) or the recently introduced optical microangiography algorithm, which is based on the absolute difference between linear intensities [3].

Topcon's novel, patent motion contrast measure uses a ratio method, named OCTARA (OCTA Ratio Analysis), in which the full spectrum is kept intact and therefore the axial resolution is preserved. Topcon's innovative method provides advantages over differentiation-based approaches while possessing improved sensitivity over methods based on amplitude decorrelation.

For OCTA processing with OCTARA, B-scan repetition at each scan location is registered. OCTA images are generated by computing a ratio-based result, r, between corresponding image pixels as follows:

$$r(x,y) = 1 - \frac{1}{N} \sum_{i,j}^{N} \frac{\min\left(I_i(x,y), I_j(x,y)\right)}{\max\left(I_i(x,y), I_j(x,y)\right)},$$

where $I(x, y)$ is the OCT signal intensity, N is the number of scanned B-scan combinations at a given location, and i and j represent two frames within any given combination of frames. This formula represents a relative measurement of OCT signal amplitude change that optimizes angiographic visualization over both the retina and choroid and also enhances the minimum detectable signal relative to amplitude decorrelation. It should be noted that the directionality of the ratio is arbitrary (i.e., numerator versus denominator) and that the subtraction from unity is an optional operation that serves to conveniently orient the direction of the display range similar to other calculation methods, such as the differentiation and decorrelation methods. Furthermore, this

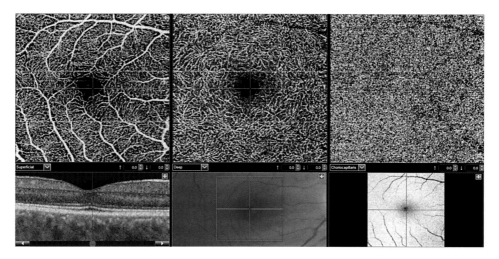

Fig. 1. *En face* optical coherence tomography (OCT) angiography (OCTA) image of the macula obtained using Topcon's IMAGEnet® 6 software, showing the superficial (top left) and deep (top center) capillary plexuses as well as the choriocapillaris (top right) using the default settings. The corresponding OCT cross section (bottom left), infrared reflectance fundus image (bottom center), and *en face* OCT image (bottom right) are also shown.

method preserves the integrity of the entire spectrum and therefore does not result in compromised axial resolution, an inherent disadvantage of split-spectrum OCTA techniques. Motion artifacts were suppressed by selectively averaging multiple B-scan combinations in the present OCTA study. High-quality OCT structural images were generated by averaging registered B-scans. Segmentation of retinal layer boundaries was performed on OCT structural images.

Standard OCT structural imaging provides intensity images for the evaluation of retinal structure and anatomy. Functional OCTA imaging detects motion by measuring intensity fluctuations in repeatedly scanned OCT images and enables visualization of blood flow and microvasculature physiology. Since OCTA is processed using OCT intensity images, the functional data are intrinsically registered with the structural data.

En face projections of volumetric scans allow for visualization of structural and vascular details within segmented retinal layer boundaries.

Comprehensive structural and functional imaging of the human retina was performed by standard OCT and OCTA. In the foveal region of a normal eye, the retinal vasculature and foveal avascular zone were clearly visualized. The inner vascular plexus in the ganglion cell layer and an outer layer of capillaries in the inner nuclear layer were readily distinguishable. The densely packed choriocapillaris network was also detected (fig. 1, macula 3 × 3). In the optic nerve head region, the radial peripapillary capillary network and microcirculation in the disk were visualized (fig. 2, OD 3 × 3).

Topcon's innovative OCTA processing method, OCTARA, which is based on a ratio calculation, demonstrates improved detection sensitivity of microvasculature. In figure 3, note that the vascular network is better visualized compared to that observed using the split-spectrum amplitude-decorrelation angiography algorithm [2]. In this example, it should be noted that the differences in relative angiographic signal intensity are due to the separate factors for both full-spectrum

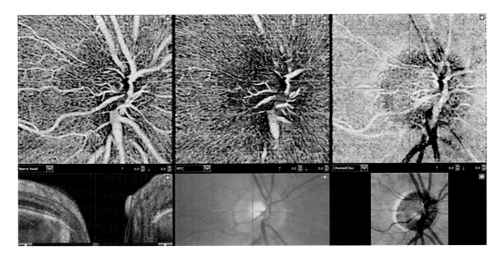

Fig. 2. *En face* OCTA image of the optic nerve head obtained using Topcon's IMAGEnet® 6 software, showing the superficial vascular layers (top left), emphasizing the radial peripapillary network (top center), and the deep vascular layers (top right) using the default settings. The corresponding OCT cross section (bottom left), color fundus image (bottom center), and *en face* OCT image (bottom right) are also shown.

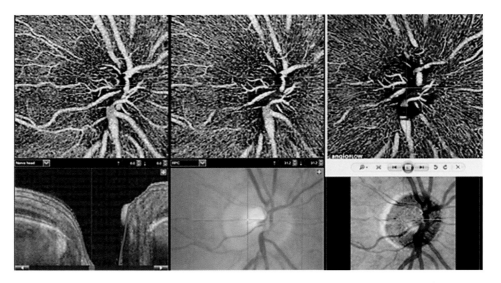

Fig. 3. *En face* OCTA image of the optic nerve head obtained using Topcon's IMAGEnet® 6 software, showing the superficial vascular layers (top left), emphasizing the radial peripapillary network (top center), using the default settings. A similar OCTA image was generated using the split-spectrum amplitude-decorrelation angiography algorithm for comparison (top right). The corresponding OCT cross section (bottom left), color fundus image (bottom center), and *en face* OCT image (bottom right) are also shown.

versus split-spectrum techniques and ratio versus amplitude decorrelation. The effects of these two sets of factors are additive in nature.

Together with industry-leading, high-speed, 1 μm-wavelength, high-tissue-penetration SS-OCT, Topcon's OCTARA method can facilitate better visualization and detailed evaluation of the individual capillary layers as well as the choroidal vasculature.

References

1 Mariampillai A, Standish BA, Moriyama EH, Khurana M, Munce NR, Leung MK, Jiang J, Cable A, Wilson BC, Vitkin IA, Yang VX: Speckle variance detection of microvasculature using swept-source optical coherence tomography. Opt Lett 2008;33:1530–1532.

2 Jia Y, Tan O, Tokayer J, Potsaid B, Wang Y, Liu JJ, Kraus MF, Subhash H, Fujimoto JG, Hornegger J, Huang D: Split-spectrum amplitude-decorrelation angiography with optical coherence tomography. Opt Express 2012;20:4710–4725.

3 Huang Y, Zhang Q, Thorell MR, An L, Durbin MK, Laron M, Sharma U, Gregori G, Rosenfeld PJ, Wang RK: Swept-source OCT angiography of the retinal vasculature using intensity differentiation-based optical microangiography algorithms. Ophthalmic Surg Lasers Imaging Retina 2014;45:382–389.

Paulo E. Stanga
Manchester Vision Regeneration (MVR) Lab
Research Office, Purple Zone, MRI
Central Manchester University Hospitals NHS
Foundation Trust
Oxford Road
Manchester M13 9WL (UK)
E-Mail Paulo.Stanga@cmft.nhs.uk

Bandello F, Souied EH, Querques G (eds): OCT Angiography in Retinal and Macular Diseases.
Dev Ophthalmol. Basel, Karger, 2016, vol 56, pp 18–29 (DOI: 10.1159/000442773)

ZEISS Angioplex™ Spectral Domain Optical Coherence Tomography Angiography: Technical Aspects

Philip J. Rosenfeld[a] · Mary K. Durbin[b] · Luiz Roisman[a] · Fang Zheng[a] · Andrew Miller[a] · Gillian Robbins[a] · Karen B. Schaal[a] · Giovanni Gregori[a]

[a]Department of Ophthalmology, Bascom Palmer Eye Institute, University of Miami Miller School of Medicine, Miami, FL, and
[b]Advanced Development, Carl Zeiss Meditec, Inc., Dublin, CA, USA

Abstract

ZEISS Angioplex™ optical coherence tomography (OCT) angiography generates high-resolution three-dimensional maps of the retinal and choroidal microvasculature while retaining all of the capabilities of the existing CIRRUS™ HD-OCT Model 5000 instrument. Angioplex™ OCT angiographic imaging on the CIRRUS™ HD-OCT platform was made possible by increasing the scanning rate to 68,000 A-scans per second and introducing improved tracking software known as FastTrac™ retinal-tracking technology. The generation of *en face* microvascular flow images with Angioplex™ OCT uses an algorithm known as OCT microangiography-complex, which incorporates differences in both the phase and intensity information contained within sequential B-scans performed at the same position. Current scanning patterns for *en face* angiographic visualization include a 3 × 3 and a 6 × 6 mm scan pattern on the retina. A volumetric dataset showing erythrocyte flow information can then be displayed as a color-coded retinal depth map in which the microvasculature of the superficial, deep, and avascular layers of the retina are displayed together with the colors red, representing the superficial microvasculature; green, representing the deep retinal vasculature; and blue, representing any vessels present in the normally avascular outer retina. Each retinal layer can be viewed separately, and the microvascular layers representing the choriocapillaris and the remaining choroid can be viewed separately as well. In addition, readjusting the contours of the slabs to target different layers of interest can generate custom *en face* flow images. Moreover, each *en face* flow image is accompanied by an *en face* intensity image to help with the interpretation of the flow results. Current clinical experience with this technology would suggest that OCT angiography should replace fluorescein angiography for retinovascular diseases involving any area of the retina that can be currently scanned with the CIRRUS™ HD-OCT instrument and may replace fluorescein angiography and indocyanine green angiography for some choroidal vascular diseases.

© 2016 S. Karger AG, Basel

Introduction

The ZEISS HD-OCT Model 5000 instrument with Angioplex™ optical coherence tomography (OCT) angiography capability is an upgrade of the existing CIRRUS™ Model 5000 instrument

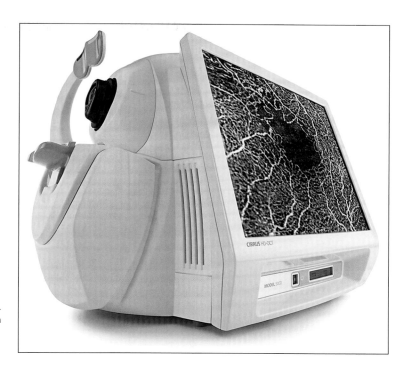

Fig. 1. Image of ZEISS HD-OCT Model 5000 instrument with Angioplex™ optical coherence tomography angiography capability.

(fig. 1). This spectral domain OCT instrument, now capable of scanning at a rate of 68,000 A-scans per second, continues to use a superluminescent diode (center wavelength of 840 nm and bandwidth of 90 nm) as its optical source, with an A-scan depth of 2.0 mm in tissue (1,024 pixels), an axial resolution of 5 microns in tissue and a transverse resolution of 15 microns. In addition, the Model 5000 incorporates Angioplex™ OCT angiography capability for noninvasive depth-encoded imaging of the retinal and choroidal microvasculature. The angiographic images are generated using a complex algorithm that analyzes differences in both intensity and phase information from repeated B-scans at the same position. This process is repeated at multiple adjacent positions to generate an *en face* flow volume. The algorithm used to generate these flow images from repeated B-scans is known as OCT microangiography-complex (OMAG^C). ZEISS Angioplex™ OCT imaging also incorporates FastTrac™ reti-

nal-tracking technology to achieve three-dimensional *en face* angiographic images with minimal movement artifacts, and FastTrac™ is also a feature of the latest CIRRUS™ HD-OCT Model 5000. This technology uses multiple channels of concurrent imaging and proprietary algorithms to monitor and correct for the motion of the eye in real time. During the scanning process, the retina is sampled at 15 frames per second to ensure that the effects of motion are significantly reduced. By only re-scanning selective data that might be affected by motion, FastTrac™ ensures faster data acquisition. Moreover, FastTrac™ also allows precise scanning at follow-up visits so that data are acquired at the same position on the retina.

The current ZEISS CIRRUS™ HD-OCT Model 5000 with Angioplex™ OCT angiography capability has all of the functionalities of the standard CIRRUS™ instrument. This instrument is capable of performing all of the intensity-based

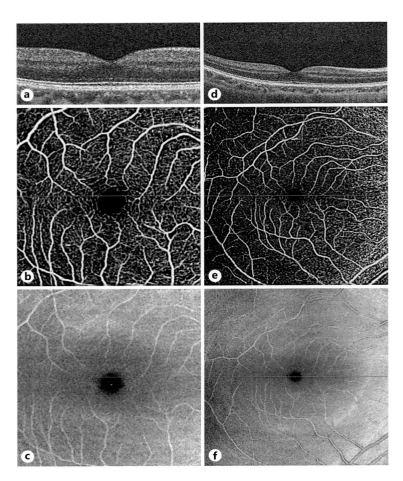

Fig. 2. Normal retina. *En face* flow images and intensity-based structural images of the superficial retinal layer along with representative B-scans that contain the boundary segmentation lines of the slab.
a–c 3 × 3 mm scans. **d–f** 6 × 6 mm scans. **a, d** B-scans with segmentation lines outlining the layer.
b, e Superficial retinal layer flow image. **c, f** Superficial retinal layer intensity image.

scan patterns and has all of the *en face* imaging capabilities that are currently available on the CIRRUS™ HD-OCT Model 5000. In addition, all of the scans that are acquired using Angioplex™ imaging can also be viewed using the standard intensity-based *en face* algorithms available on the CIRRUS™. The user can visualize B-scan images and *en face* or partial *en face* images of the collected data either as an intensity-based scan or an OMAG^C scan [1–4]. These volumetric datasets can then be manipulated by choosing different pre-selected surfaces to generate *en face* images or by choosing slabs with different contours so that custom *en face* images can be generated. The user

can then manipulate the boundaries of these slabs to optimize the visualization of pathology in different anatomic layers.

The standard scanning patterns that are available when using ZEISS Angioplex™ OCT angiography include cube scans of 3 × 3 and 6 × 6 mm. To image vascular flow, each B-scan in the scan pattern is consecutively repeated several times. Comparisons of intensity and phase information from consecutive B-scans in the same location will reveal some areas that undergo changes over time and some areas without change. Temporal differences with respect to both intensity and phase information at a specific location are

Rosenfeld · Durbin · Roisman · Zheng · Miller · Robbins · Schaal · Gregori

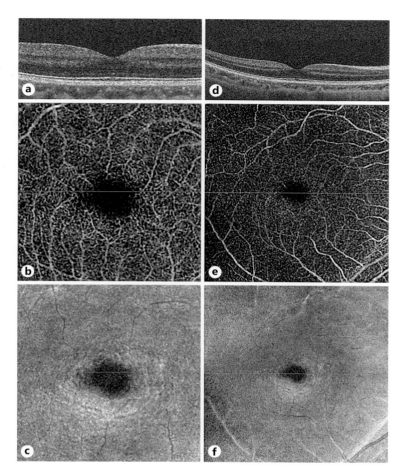

Fig. 3. Normal retina. *En face* flow images and intensity-based structural images of the deep retinal layer along with representative B-scans that contain the boundary segmentation lines of the slab. **a–c** 3 × 3 mm scans. **d–f** 6 × 6 mm scans. **a, d** B-scans with segmentation lines outlining the layer. **b, e** Deep retinal layer flow image. **c, f** Deep retinal layer intensity image.

principally due to erythrocyte motion and indicate the location of a vessel. OMAG^C analysis of all B-scans along a cube results in the mapping of the location of blood flow in three dimensions throughout the scanned area.

When the 3 × 3 mm scan pattern is used, there are 245 A-scans in each B-scan along the horizontal dimension and 245 B-scan positions long the vertical dimension. As a result, each A-scan and B-scan is separated by 12.2 microns. When an OCT angiographic image is acquired using the 3 × 3 mm scan pattern, each B-scan is repeated four times at the same position. When using the 6 × 6 mm scan pattern, each B-scan contains 350 A-scans equally spaced along the horizontal dimension so that there is a separation of 17.1 microns between A-scans. Similarly, there are 350 B-scan positions in the vertical direction, and each B-scan is separated by 17.1 microns. Each B-scan in the 6 × 6 mm scan is repeated twice at the same position.

For each of the scan patterns, B-scan and *en face* structural images are generated along with three-dimensional microvascular maps of the retinal and choroidal circulation. The instrument provides settings for default *en face* images of both the retinal and choroidal vasculature, but boundary layers can be manipulated to provide

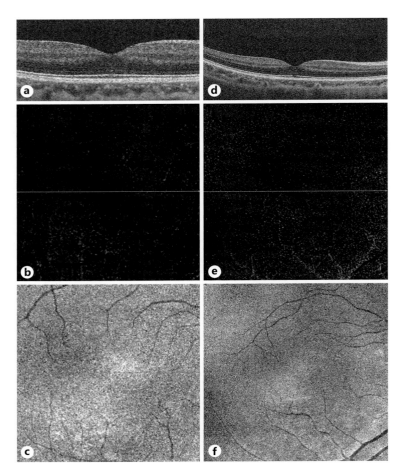

Fig. 4. Normal retina. *En face* flow images and intensity-based structural images of the avascular retinal layer along with representative B-scans that contain the boundary segmentation lines of the slab. **a–c** 3 × 3 mm scans. **d–f** 6 × 6 mm scans. **a, d** B-scans with segmentation lines outlining the layer. **b, e** Avascular retinal layer flow image. **c, f** Avascular layer intensity image.

custom layers that depict the microvasculature between those chosen boundaries. The standard contour maps for retinal segmentation use the internal limiting membrane (ILM) as the inner contour and the segmentation of the retinal pigment epithelium (RPE) as the outer contour. The thickness between these two contours is provided as an optional overlay on either the angiographic *en face* or the structural *en face* images with adjustable transparency. This allows the detection of edema and other typical effects observed on an OCT thickness map. The retina is subdivided into additional layers, and the ILM contour is used as the inner boundary and the RPE contour is used

as the outer boundary of these additional layers. The innermost layer or slab is referred to as the superficial retinal layer, which extends from the ILM to the inner plexiform layer. In a normal retina, this layer would include the superficial capillary plexus (fig. 2). The deep capillary plexus is found in the deep retinal layer, which extends from the inner nuclear layer to the outer plexiform layer (fig. 3). The avascular layer extends from 110 microns above the RPE to 60 microns above the RPE. This avascular slab was constructed with the goal of bounding the parts of the retina that are expected to have no vasculature in normal anatomy (fig. 4). There are many

Rosenfeld · Durbin · Roisman · Zheng · Miller · Robbins · Schaal · Gregori

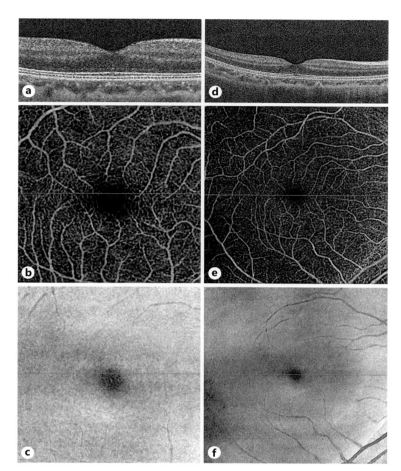

Fig. 5. Normal retina. *En face* flow images and intensity-based structural images of a total retina color-coded depth flow map along with representative B-scans that contain the boundary segmentation lines of the slab. **a–c** 3 × 3 mm scans. **d–f** 6 × 6 mm scans. **a, d** B-scans with segmentation lines outlining the layer. **b, e** Total retina color-coded depth flow image. **c, f** Total retina intensity image.

situations for which there may appear to be bright areas in this image that are not necessarily due to pathology, such as artifacts from the overlying flow signals and errors in segmentation, which are particularly common in the presence of geographic atrophy, or nonflow-related pathologies, such as exudates and the presence of hyper-reflective foci, which are thought to represent dissociated RPE. If there is flow and abnormally appearing microvasculature in the avascular slab, then the segmentation lines and the corresponding structural B-scans and *en face* images should be examined carefully to ensure that the flow represents true pathology. The total retina color-coded depth map represents the entire retinal vasculature. The microvasculature within the superficial retinal layer is depicted in red, the microvasculature in the deep retinal layer is represented by green, and any detectable flow in the avascular retinal layer is represented by blue (fig. 5).

A slab that extends from 29 microns beneath the RPE to 49 microns beneath the RPE best represents the default choriocapillaris layer, and the contour of this layer follows the RPE segmentation boundary layer (fig. 6). The choroidal layer is represented by a slab that follows the contour of the RPE-Fit line, which is segmented as described in the chapter on advanced visualization

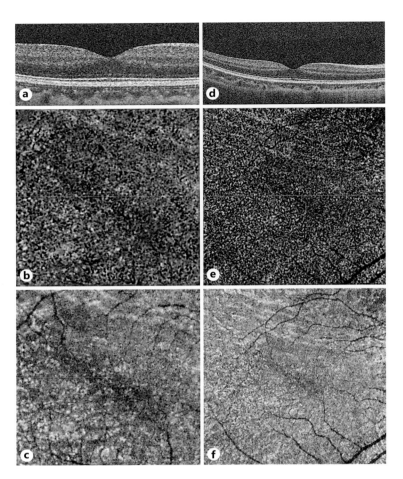

Fig. 6. Normal retina. *En face* flow images and intensity-based structural images of the choriocapillaris layer along with representative B-scans that contain the boundary segmentation lines of the slab. **a–c** 3 × 3 mm scans. **d–f** 6 × 6 mm scans. **a, d** B-scans with segmentation lines outlining the layer. **b, e** Choriocapillaris layer flow image. **c, f** Choriocapillaris layer intensity image.

that can be found in the user's manual. This RPE-Fit line is intended as an estimate of the Bruch's membrane (BM). The choroidal layer has a uniform thickness of 51 microns and is represented by a slab that extends from 64 microns to 115 microns below the RPE-Fit line or BM (fig. 7).

The positions of the boundaries for all layers and the thicknesses of the layers can be manipulated, and *en face* images of both the microvasculature flow information and the structural information that correspond to these adjusted slabs are generated in real time. Moreover, a custom feature is available in which different inner and outer

boundary contours can be chosen, and their positions can be manipulated to optimize the *en face* visualization of the retinal and choroidal microvasculature, as well as their corresponding structural images.

Additional slabs include a whole retina *en face* image, which is intended to illustrate the vasculature of the entire retina. The inner boundary of this image is the ILM. The outer boundary is offset by 60 microns above the RPE in order to minimize the contribution of the hyper-reflective RPE. There is also a whole eye *en face* image, which sums all of the flow signals within an entire scan volume. This image may be useful when

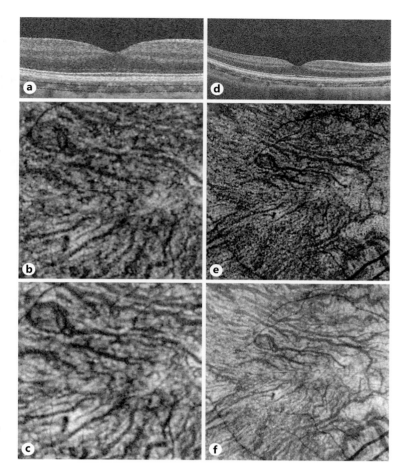

Fig. 7. Normal retina. *En face* flow images and intensity-based structural images of the choroidal layer along with representative B-scans that contain the boundary segmentation lines of the slab. **a–c** 3 × 3 mm scans. **d–f** 6 × 6 mm scans. **a, d** B-scans with segmentation lines outlining the layer. **b, e** Choroidal layer flow image. **c, f** Choroidal layer intensity image.

segmentation failures occur due to anatomic distortions caused by disease and the best *en face* flow image is obtained by viewing the entire scan. There is also an *en face* image that illustrates the vasculature that appears above the retina. The boundaries of this *en face* image extend from the vitreoretinal interface to 300 microns above the interface. Finally, the software offers the possibility of overlaying either the flow image or the structural *en face* image with the thickness map, which allows the user to evaluate when edema is present.

To help with the interpretation of the flow images from each of the *en face* images, the algo-rithm provides a corresponding *en face* structural image with each *en face* flow image. This structural image is useful for assessing the strength of signal intensity. If the flow signal in any *en face* image appears absent or reduced, then the corresponding intensity image needs to be viewed to determine if the flow is really compromised or whether the intensity signal is diminished. If the intensity signal is diminished, then it is impossible to make any conclusion about whether flow is present, decreased, or simply undetectable due to the absence of an intensity signal. Perhaps the loss of the signal is due to increased light scattering from an overlying layer, resulting in de-

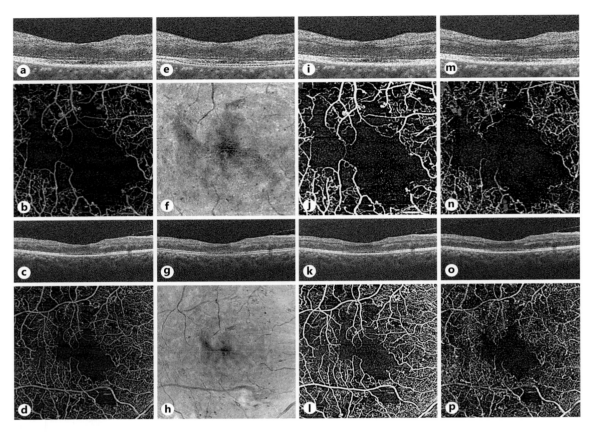

Fig. 8. Diabetic retina. *En face* total retina color-coded depth flow map, total retina intensity map, superficial retinal layer flow images, and deep retinal layer flow images. **a** 3 mm horizontal B-scan through fovea corresponding to **b**. **b** 3 × 3 mm total retina color-coded depth flow map. **c** 6 mm horizontal B-scan scan through fovea corresponding to **d**. **d** 6 × 6 mm scan total retina color-coded depth flow map. **e** 3 mm horizontal B-scan through fovea with segmentation lines outlining the total retinal intensity layer shown in **f**. **f** 3 × 3 mm total retinal intensity image. **g** 6 mm horizontal B-scan through fovea with segmentation lines outlining the total retinal intensity layer shown in **h**. **h** 6 × 6 mm total retinal intensity image. **i** 3 mm horizontal B-scan through fovea with segmentation lines outlining the superficial retinal layer shown in **j**. **j** 3 × 3 mm superficial retinal layer flow image. **k** 6 mm horizontal B-scan through fovea with segmentation lines outlining the superficial retinal layer shown in **l**. **l** 6 × 6 mm superficial retinal layer flow image. **m** 3 mm horizontal B-scan through fovea with segmentation lines outlining the deep retinal layer shown in **n**. **n** 3 × 3 mm deep retinal layer flow image. **o** 6 mm horizontal B-scan through fovea with segmentation lines outlining the deep retinal layer shown in **p**. **p** 6 × 6 mm deep retinal layer flow image.

creased light penetration into the retina or choroid with the subsequent loss of a signal in the layer. The decreased signal would then erroneously appear as an apparent decrease in flow, but it would be an artifact that results from the loss of signal rather than a real decrease in flow. What-

ever the reason, the intensity *en face* image is crucial for the appropriate interpretation of the *en face* flow image.

Representative Angioplex™ OCT angiography images of diabetic retinopathy, macular telangiectasia type 2, and choroidal neovascular-

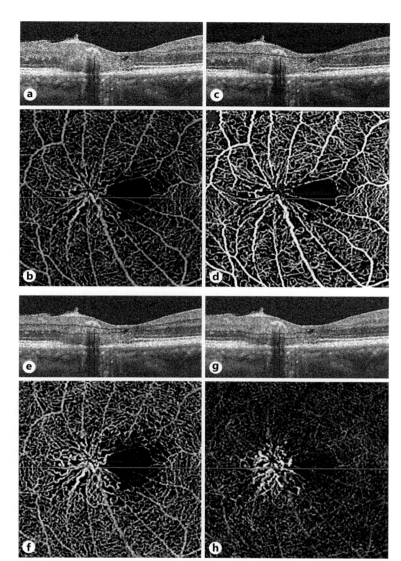

Fig. 9. Macular telangiectasia type 2. *En face* total retina color-coded depth flow image, superficial retinal layer flow image, deep retinal layer flow image, and avascular retinal layer flow image (3 × 3 mm scans). **a**, **c**, **e**, **g** B-scans with segmentation lines outlining the layer. **b** *En face* total retina color-coded depth flow image. **d** Superficial retinal layer flow image. **f** Deep retinal layer flow image. **h** Avascular retinal layer flow map.

ization from age-related macular degeneration are shown in figures 8 through 10. Figure 8 shows a diabetic retina with a loss of normal macular microvasculature along with the appearance of microaneurysms. Both the 3 × 3 and the 6 × 6 mm images of the total, superficial, and deep retinal layers show evidence of decreased microvascular flow within the macula. The corresponding intensity images of the total retinal layer confirm that the diminished flow in the retina is real and not due to the loss of the signal intensity. Figure 9 shows a case of advanced macular telangiectasia type 2 with distortion of the perifoveal microvasculature and temporal anastomoses between retinal layers. The color-coding of the total retinal flow *en face* image shows color-encoded depth information that reveals abnormal communications between the

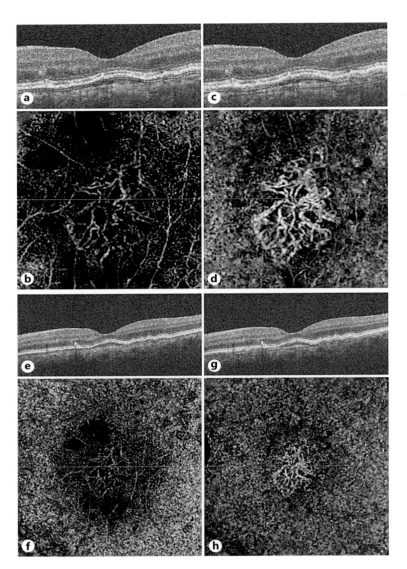

Fig. 10. Neovascular age-related macular degeneration. *En face* choriocapillaris layer flow image and custom map flow image. **a–d** 3 × 3 mm scans. **e–h** 6 × 6 mm scans. **a, c, e, g** B-scans with segmentation lines outlining the layer. **b, f** Choriocapillaris layer flow image. **d, h** Custom segmentation flow image with the retinal pigment epithelium as the contour of the inner boundary and the RPE-Fit line (Bruch's membrane) as the contour of the outer boundary.

superficial, deep, and avascular retinal layers. The individual layers that comprise the whole retinal blood flow image are also shown. Figure 10 shows type 1 neovascularization in age-related macular degeneration imaged using the choriocapillaris layer generated by Angioplex™ OCT angiography. However, the best visualization of the neovascularization is observed by using the custom map in which the RPE layer serves as one boundary contour and the RPE-Fit line (BM) serves at the outer boundary contour, with the thickness of the layer adjusted to optimize the signal intensity from the neovascular complex. This technology is remarkable for its ease of use and ability to provide information about the three-dimensional structure of the retinal and choroidal microvasculature.

Summary

ZEISS Angioplex™ OCT angiography is a fast, safe, noninvasive, easily repeatable method for generating high-quality images of the retinal and choroidal microvasculature. This new platform incorporates all of the capabilities of the Cirrus HD-OCT Model 5000 instrument along with an increased scan rate of 68,000 A-scans per second and FastTrac™ retinal-tracking technology for motion correction and reproducible follow-up positioning of scans. Two different scan patterns covering a 3×3 and a 6×6 mm region of the retina are available along with proprietary segmentation algorithms that permit layer-by-layer visualization of the retinal and choroidal microvasculature. Angioplex™ OCT angiography provides better imaging of the retinal microvasculature compared with conventional fluorescein angiography (FA), and this technology can image the choriocapillaris better than conventional indocyanine green angiography. While OCT angiography is unable to detect active leakage, pooling or staining from the microvasculature, active leakage can still be inferred by using conventional OCT imaging to detect increased retinal thickening, and these structural images are still available as part of the routine Angioplex™ image analysis package. Although it should be noted that CIRRUS Angioplex™ is not currently indicated as a substitute for FA, our clinical experience to date with this technology suggests that OCT angiography may be able to replace FA for retinovascular diseases involving any area that can be scanned with the CIRRUS™ HD-OCT and may replace FA and indocyanine green angiography for some choroidal microvascular diseases.

Disclosures

Dr. Rosenfeld and Dr. Gregori receive research support from Carl Zeiss Meditec. Dr. Rosenfeld also receives research support from Acucela, Apellis, Genentech/Roche, GlaxoSmithKline, Neurotech, Ocata Therapeutics, and Tyrogenex. He is a consultant for Achillion, Acucela, Alcon, Bayer, Chengdu Kanghong Biotech, CoDa Therapeutics, Genentech/Roche, Healios K.K., Merck, Regeneron, Stealth, and Tyrogenex.

Dr. Durbin is an employee of Carl Zeiss Meditec, Inc.

Dr. Gregori and the University of Miami co-own a patent that is licensed to Carl Zeiss Meditec, Inc.

References

1 Huang Y, Zhang Q, Thorell MR, An L, Durbin MK, Laron M, et al: Swept-source OCT angiography of the retinal vasculature using intensity differentiation-based optical microangiography algorithms. Ophthalmic Surg Lasers Imaging Retina 2014;45:382–389.

2 Reif R, Baran U, Wang RK: Motion artifact and background noise suppression on optical microangiography frames using a naive Bayes mask. Appl Opt 2014;53:4164–4171.

3 Thorell MR, Zhang Q, Huang Y, An L, Durbin MK, Laron M, et al: Swept-source OCT angiography of macular telangiectasia type 2. Ophthalmic Surg Lasers Imaging Retina 2014;45:369–380.

4 Zhang Q, Wang RK, Chen CL, Legarreta AD, Durbin MK, An L, et al: Swept-source OCT angiography of neovascular macular telangiectasia type 2. Ophthalmic Surg Lasers Imaging Retina 2015; 45:369.

Philip J. Rosenfeld, MD, PhD
Bascom Palmer Eye Institute
900 NW 17th Street
Miami, FL 33136 (USA)
E-Mail prosenfeld@miami.edu

Bandello F, Souied EH, Querques G (eds): OCT Angiography in Retinal and Macular Diseases.
Dev Ophthalmol. Basel, Karger, 2016, vol 56, pp 30–36 (DOI: 10.1159/000442774)

Image Analysis of Optical Coherence Tomography Angiography

Gabriel Coscas[a, b] • Marco Lupidi[a, c] • Florence Coscas[a, b]

[a]Centre de l'Odéon, Paris, and [b]Department of Ophthalmology, Centre Hospitalier Intercommunal de Créteil, Université Paris Est, Créteil, France; [c]Department of Biomedical and Surgical Sciences, Section of Ophthalmology, University of Perugia, S. Maria della Misericordia Hospital, Perugia, Italy

Abstract

Optical coherence tomography (OCT) angiography (OCT-A) is a transformative approach in imaging ocular vessels based on flow rather than simple reflectance intensity. It is therefore a functional extension of OCT that can be used to visualize microvasculature by detecting motion contrast from flowing blood. As OCT-A is a depth-resolved examination, it needs careful axial segmentation in order to preserve important data on perfused structures and to avoid the risk of generating superimposed images, which are typical of dye angiographies. An *automated segmentation algorithm* for both retinal and choroidal layers is provided by the majority of different OCT-A devices. In the case of accentuated macular retinal/choroidal disruptions causing potential segmentation errors, specific manual correction allows one to modify the shape and the localization of each layer. In the case of *manual segmentation,* the thickness of every C-scan may be modified in order to provide a constant thickness of tissue slices at different retinal or choroidal levels. OCT projection artifacts also occur from superficial retinal vessels, which can be seen in deeper retinal layers, or retinal and choroidal vessels, which can even be seen in the scleral tissue. These projection artifacts are almost always present and are visible in any layer that is located below the perfused vasculature. © 2016 S. Karger AG, Basel

Introduction

Optical coherence tomography (OCT) angiography (OCT-A) is a transformative approach for imaging ocular vessels based on flow rather than simple reflectance intensity. It is therefore a functional extension of OCT that can be used to visualize microvasculature by detecting motion contrast from flowing blood.

The basis of OCT-A is to repeatedly scan a region and then examine the resultant images for changes. Stationary tissue structures will show lit-

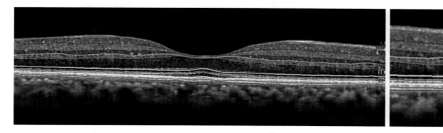

Fig. 1. Automated segmentation algorithm. Eleven different layers are identified by automatic segmentation. These layers represent the inner limiting membrane (ILM), the retinal nerve fiber layer, the ganglion cell layer, the inner plexiform layer, the inner nuclear layer, the outer plexiform layer, the external limiting membrane, the ellipsoid zone, the outer segment, the retinal pigment epithelium and *Bruch's membrane*. The possibility of obtaining precise distinction between the different layers is a useful function both in conventional and in angiographic modes and allows one to easily define the localization and axial extension of a given lesion, as well as the presence of a perfused structure within the examined tissue.

tle change, whereas moving structures, such as blood flowing through vessels, can show changes between images.

Because there are many ways to measure an image (e.g. speckle or intensity decorrelation, phase variance, etc.), there are ultimately many ways to look for flow. Each of these methods has advantages and disadvantages, and all of them depend on the quality and limits of the original OCT images.

The resultant image looks like an angiogram but is derived only from signals intrinsically generated from tissue, without the need for contrast agent injection. This imaging technique can be performed rapidly and repeatedly, potentially at every patient visit, as well as in patients for whom fluorescein angiography (FA) or indocyanine green angiography may not be indicated.

OCT-A can be used to visualize both retinal vessels and vessels under the retinal pigment epithelium (RPE) and provides depth-resolved images. Despite these advantages, OCT-A images can have many types of artifacts, which are important to recognize when interpreting images.

As OCT-A is a depth-resolved examination, it needs careful axial segmentation in order to preserve important data on perfused structures and to avoid the risk of generating superimposed images, which are typical of dye angiographies.

How to Segment an Optical Coherence Tomography Angiogram

Depth-resolved OCT analysis can be achieved through either automated or manual layer segmentation.

An *automated segmentation algorithm* for both retinal and choroidal layers is provided by the majority of different OCT-A devices (fig. 1).

This algorithm is capable of distinguishing several different retinal layers, from the inner limiting membrane (ILM) to the RPE, including the external limiting membrane, ellipsoid zone and outer segment. The possibility of obtaining precise distinction between different layers is a useful function of conventional mode because it allows one to easily define the axial extension of a given lesion in retinal tissue.

Moreover, OCT-A acquires an essential role because it rapidly shows exact morpho-functional correspondence: a given decorrelation signal due to a perfused structure can be topographically localized. As the vascular and avascular layers are well known, the presence (or absence) of perfusion in a location may significantly help in distinguishing a normal condition from an abnormal one, aiding not only in diagnosis but also in treatment decision.

In the case of accentuated macular retinal/choroidal disruptions causing potential segmentation errors, specific manual correction allows one to modify the shape and the localization of each layer.

In case of *manual segmentation*, the thickness of every C-scan may be modified in order to provide a constant tissue slice thickness at different retinal or choroidal levels. Therefore, this approach allows detailed analysis of all of the structures included in a certain 'slab of tissue' obtained in 'en face' visualization.

The manual selection of C-scans at different depths may be performed with either horizontal or variably shaped sections. A horizontal section (not aligned to any retinal layer) might be chosen with the aim of reducing artifacts due to segmentation errors.

Different shapes, according to our experience, may be chosen based on several parameters.

First, in the presence of segmentation errors, when the profile of a C-scan is not perfectly aligned to the structure taken as a reference (i.e. ILM, RPE, or Bruch's membrane [BM]), it is better to avoid this approach in order to avoid the risk of superimposition or missing structures in the C-scan.

Second, it is important to consider the layer or the lesion that will be analyzed. For example, when imaging a choroidal neovascularization lesion, it might be important to obtain a C-scan shaped on the RPE profile, as neovascular tissue is often attached to the back surface of the pigmented epithelium.

Finally, the concavity or convexity of a scanned area should be considered. In some conditions, such as high myopia or dome-shaped macula, a section aligned on the RPE or BM may be more suitable than a horizontal one, as the latter would show different structures (from one to the other) in the same C-scan.

In the case of retinal vascular disease, such as artery/vein occlusion or diabetic retinopathy, it is important to analyze the entire retinal thickness. This procedure is necessary not only to have a comprehensive assessment of the scanned tissue but also to exclude potential artifacts, which might affect the diagnostic process.

Therefore, mostly in the case of nonautomated segmentation, a selected C-scan should be manually fine-tuned to be located at the level of the ILM and then moved progressively deeper, with steps corresponding to the same thickness of the section, up to the RPE. In case of simultaneous outer retinal or RPE/BM changes, the entire choroidal thickness (up to the choroidal-scleral interface) should be evaluated.

Layer Segmentation in Optical Coherence Tomography Angiography

En face OCT-A images provide information about flow detected in a C-scan (i.e. en face) section.

To visualize blood flow in different retinal and choroidal anatomic layers, the layered structures have to be identified and *segmented*.

C-scan sections of variable thickness may be selected. These sections can be moved to different depths within an OCT volume scan in order to analyze the entirety of the retinal and choroidal tissue within the scanned area. Accurate layer segmentation is crucial to produce reliable OCT-A images (obtained with high-resolution OCT B-scans).

Automated layer segmentation is useful to the clinician because it provides an extremely fast way to delineate the presence of a decorrelation signal due to perfused vascular structures in any OCT-A image (fig. 2).

Fig. 2. Automated segmentation in optical coherence tomography angiography (OCT-A). **a** Superficial capillary plexus shown in C-scan OCT-A visualization. This vascular layer is typically identified at the level of the ganglion cell layer in the macular area. In both OCT-A (**b**) and conventional OCT (**c**), B-scans show the exact level at which the C-scan (**a**) is taken. **d** Deep capillary plexus shown in C-scan OCT-A visualization. This vascular layer is typically identified at the level of the inner nuclear layer. In both OCT-A (**e**) and conventional OCT (**f**), B-scans show the exact level at which the C-scan (**a**) is taken.

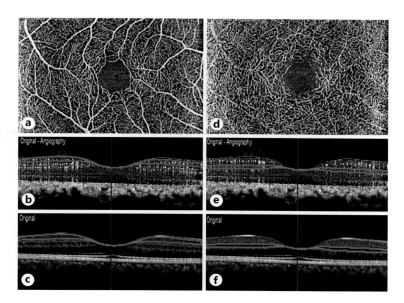

Such automated segmentation is based on the different levels of reflectivity that are visible mainly on conventional OCT B-scans. Each retinal layer is clearly distinguished from the others due to a different degree of reflectivity, which allows the identification of its borders.

Histopathologic findings allocate the retinal superficial capillary plexus to the ganglion cell layer and the deep capillary plexus to the inner nuclear layer.

Automatically segmented C-scan sections of an OCT-A image are therefore taken at the reported exact histological site and guided by conventional OCT.

As there are no clear boundaries between the different choroidal layers (e.g. the choriocapillaris, Settler's layer, and Haller's layer), the distinction is commonly made by taking into account the mean thickness of each layer (based on OCT and histopathologic findings) as well as the vessel's diameter, which is clearly visible on enhanced depth imaging OCT.

Although automated segmentation allows prompt analysis of different vascular layers, it can suffer from *potential segmentation errors*.

These errors especially occur in accentuated macular diseases, which significantly alter the profile and the reflectivity of the neuro-retina. The software in these cases might be no more capable of correctly distinguishing the borders of each retinal layer, and different layers will often converge into a single layer. These errors are cause by the fact that on C-scans several structures are shown as coplanar when in fact they belong to different layers.

Nevertheless, in the case of segmentation error, the various available OCT devices allow for the manual correction of all boundaries.

Manual segmentation allows a fully customizable analysis and is usually not much more time consuming than automated segmentation.

Manual segmentation is based on both the possibility of selecting C-scan section thickness and the shaping of a section using the most suitable profile (fig. 3).

In the case of manual processing, the thickness of every section is very important.

A thin C-scan section allows the finest details of a vascular structure to be distinguished because the risk of generating a superimposed image is minimal.

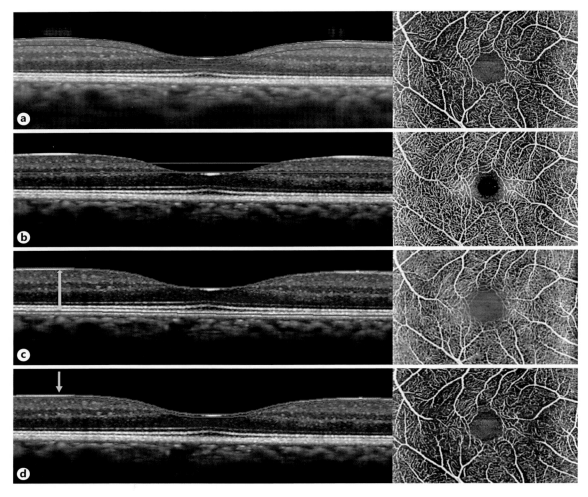

Fig. 3. Manual segmentation in OCT-A. Each figure (**a–d**) shows the manual selection of the shape and thickness of a section on conventional OCT (left) and the corresponding image in C-scan visualization (right). **a** A 50-μm-thick section aligned on the ILM profile. The conventional B-scan OCT image shows the exact localization of the section (left). On the right, the resulting C-scan OCT-A image is shown. **b** A 50-μm-thick horizontal section (right) and corresponding C-scan in angiographic mode (left). **c** A thick section (yellow double-arrow) that includes the entire neuro-retina between the ILM and the retinal pigment epithelium. The two profiles bordering the section are shaped on the ILM and ellipsoid zone profiles. Such a thick section might be useful when comparing OCT-A with conventional fluorescein angiography, as both examination techniques show all vascular layers as superimposed. **d** Thin section (yellow arrow) shaped on the ILM profile. This approach is useful for distinguishing the finest details of a vascular structure.

Conversely, a thick section might still be useful to analyze a certain layer or lesion over its entire thickness. Moreover, a thick section is the most suitable choice to compare a given OCT-A image to one generated by conventional FA. FA is a bi-dimensional examination technique in which all structures are overlapped. A thick section might be used to assimilate OCT-A, which offers a three-dimensional, depth-resolved exam and is therefore comparable with conventional angiography.

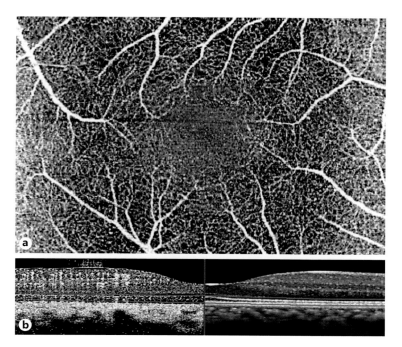

Fig. 4. Reflection artifacts in OCT-A. **a** Large retinal vessels and superficial and deep capillary plexa shown in C-scan OCT-A visualization. These vascular layers are generally located at the level of the inner retina. In both OCT-A and conventional mode, B-scans (**b**) show that the corresponding C-scan (**a**) is segmented at the level of the outer retina, more precisely between the external limiting membrane and Bruch's membrane. This is therefore a typical example of a reflection artifact, which should be always taken into account when segmenting below a perfused vascular layer.

The selection of a profile for the shape of a C-scan section significantly impacts the aspect of the obtained image. In our experience, the most frequently used profiles are those of the ILM, RPE and BM. Because of their high reflectivity, these profiles suffer less from potential segmentation errors.

The ILM profile is mostly used when evaluating the retinal vascular layers, while the RPE and BM profiles are useful for the outer retina and choroid (i.e. in the case of choroidal neovascularization, the neovascular tissue is frequently attached at the back surface of the RPE).

Horizontal sections are also frequently used for segmenting retinal and choroidal layers. This has the remarkable advantage of avoiding potential segmentation errors. The disadvantage, however, is a lack of alignment to the concavities or convexities of the eye. In this way, different structures, even those at different depths, appear to be coplanar.

Reflection Artifacts in Optical Coherence Tomography Angiography

Light passing through a blood vessel can be *reflected*, *refracted*, or *absorbed*. In OCT-A, a signal is obtained due to reflected light coming from moving blood cells. Nevertheless, light that has passed through moving blood also encounters tissue below the blood vessel.

Optical Coherence Tomography Angiography Projection Artifacts

When light strikes the RPE, it is reflected back to the OCT device. Light that has passed through blood vessels varies over time; therefore, the reflection of such light is detected as having a decorrelation resembling blood flow. In this way, the RPE layer might seem to possess blood vessels that have the same character as overlying retinal vessels.

This effect is described as an OCT-A projection artifact. OCT projection artifacts also occur from superficial retinal vessels, which can be seen in deeper retinal layers, or from retinal and choroidal vessels, which can be seen in scleral tissue. These projection artifacts are almost always present and are visible in any layer that is located below the perfused vasculature (fig. 4).

Conclusion

OCT-A is a promising addition to multi-modal retinal imaging. OCT-A provides functional flow information in addition to the structural details seen on regular OCT. To generate a comprehensive assessment, OCT-A associated with regular OCT scans should be simultaneously evaluated in B-scan and C-scan views.

Prof. Gabriel Coscas
Centre Hospitalier Intercommunal de Créteil
40 Avenue de Verdun
FR–94000 Créteil (France)
E-Mail gabriel.coscas@gmail.com

Bandello F, Souied EH, Querques G (eds): OCT Angiography in Retinal and Macular Diseases.
Dev Ophthalmol. Basel, Karger, 2016, vol 56, pp 37–44 (DOI: 10.1159/000442775)

Optical Coherence Tomography Angiography in Healthy Subjects

Gabriel Coscas[a, b] · Marco Lupidi[a, c] · Florence Coscas[a, b]

[a]Centre de l'Odéon, Paris, and [b]Department of Ophthalmology, Centre Hospitalier Intercommunal de Créteil, Université Paris Est, Créteil, France; [c]Department of Biomedical and Surgical Sciences, Section of Ophthalmology, University of Perugia, S. Maria della Misericordia Hospital, Perugia, Italy

Abstract

Fluorescein angiography and indocyanine green angiography provide information about normal retinal and choroidal anatomy that is nearly comparable to histological findings. These results are absolutely fundamental for the evaluation of retinal and choroidal vascular diseases and allow the clinician to define and diagnose several pathological conditions. Fluorescein angiography has become the '*gold standard*' in retinal imaging due to its capacity to allow visualization of the retinal capillary bed and its changes, particularly in the macular area. Although the fluorescence of the injected dye enables improved visualization of retinal capillaries, not all of the different layers of the retinal capillary network can be visualized using this bi-dimensional examination technique, possibly because of a light scattering phenomenon. Optical coherence tomography angiography allows depth-resolved visualization of the retinal and choroidal microvasculature by calculating the difference between static and nonstatic tissue. Given that the main moving elements in the eye fundus are contained within vessels, determining a vascular decorrelation signal enables three-dimensional visualization of the retinal and choroidal vascular network without the administration of intravenous dye and therefore reduces the risk of potential adverse events.

© 2016 S. Karger AG, Basel

Introduction

Traditional multimodal imaging techniques, such as fluorescein angiography (FA) and indocyanine green angiography, provide essential dynamic information on the perfusion of different retinal and choroidal vascular layers, including arm-to-eye transit time. Therefore, such techniques provide information about normal retinal and choroidal anatomy that is nearly comparable to histological findings [1]. These results are absolutely fundamental for the evaluation of retinal and choroidal vascular diseases and, in combination with morphological data, allow the clinician to detect disease and define a correct diagnosis.

FA has become the *'gold standard'* technique for imaging of the fundus because it is the best method for visualizing the retinal capillary bed and its changes, particularly in the macular area. Moreover, FA allows also the clinician to detect and analyze a prominent clinical sign, namely *leakage* from abnormal and/or new vessels.

Although the fluorescence of the injected dye improves the visualization of retinal capillaries, not all of the different layers of the retinal capillary network can be visualized using this bi-dimensional examination technique. FA images of the retina detail the anatomical arrangement of superficial retinal vessels, whereas deeper retinal capillaries cannot be visualized in the angiogram [2, 3].

Comparative findings suggest that the deeper capillary network in the retina is not visualized well by FA, possibly because of light scattering in the retina [4]. Therefore, even if FA is the gold standard for the visualization of retinal vessels, one of the two major retinal capillary networks does not appear to be imaged well with this technique, despite that the retina is a nearly transparent structure [5].

Optical coherence tomography angiography (OCT-A) produces clear, depth-resolved visualization of the retinal [5] and choroidal microvasculature [6] by calculating the signal decorrelation between static and nonstatic tissue.

Given that the main moving elements in the eye fundus are contained within vessels, determining a vascular decorrelation signal enables three-dimensional visualization of the retinal and choroidal vascular network [7]. Moreover, OCT-A does not require the intravenous administration of dye, thereby reducing the risk of potential adverse events [8].

Retinal and Choroidal Vascular Analysis in Healthy Subjects

Fluorescein Angiography in Healthy Subjects
The current atlas of FA images was obtained using a confocal imaging system (Spectralis HRA2,

Heidelberg Engineering, Heidelberg, Germany). This system captures only the light emitted within a predetermined plane and consequently eliminates artifacts (due to reflection and diffraction) and superimposed images.

The macular capillary bed, including the delicate perifoveal anastomotic arcade, may be visualized in cases with clear media and good contrast. This arcade can precisely delimitate the foveal avascular zone. In some rare cases, very fine and specific focusing can help distinguish differences between the superficial capillary plexus and the deep capillary plexus (DCP), and imaging them may require successive focusing. Fine structures, including pathologic conditions such as neovascularization, are clearly visualized (fig. 1).

Retinal Optical Coherence Tomography Angiography in Healthy Subjects

OCT-A examinations are performed using a Spectralis OCT-2 Angiograph prototype (Heidelberg Engineering, Heidelberg, Germany) that can acquire 85,000 A-scans per second with an axial resolution of 7 μm at an imaging depth of 1.9 mm in tissue. The ocular light power exposure is within the American National Standards Institute safety limit [9].

C-scans allow the visualization of arteries, which are clearly distinguishable from veins based on the presence of a surrounding hypo-intense halo due to the absence of efferent vessels coming directly out of the walls.

The superficial capillary plexus appears as a fine capillary network with an intense signal. The perifoveal arcade can be visualized well at 360° (fig. 2a–c).

The DCP is visible in C-scans taken at the level of the inner nuclear layer [red line in fig. 3b and c]. A dense capillary network that differs from the superficial network becomes clearly visible and develops all around the perifoveal area.

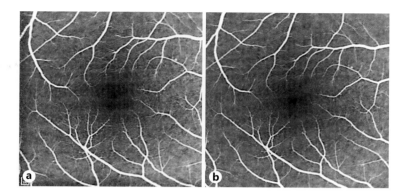

Fig. 1. Fluorescein angiography in early arteriovenous phase. **a** Both retinal veins and arteries, as well as macular branches, are fully perfused, and there is no evidence of any filling impairment. The superficial capillary plexus (SCP) is mainly visible in the perifoveal area. The perifoveal arcade is not completely appreciable. **b** Fluorescein angiography in early arterial-venous phase with a deeper focus than in (**a**) to obtain information on deep retinal vessels. The deep capillary plexus, despite the focusing process, remains unappreciable because of retinal light scattering.

Fig. 2. Visualization of the SCP. **a** Automatically obtained optical coherence tomography angiography (OCT-A) C-scan, which exactly outlines the ganglion cell layer profile (as shown in **b**, **c**). Arteries are clearly distinguishable from veins by the presence of a surrounding hypo-intense halo due to the absence of efferent vessels coming directly out of the walls. A fine capillary network, which corresponds to the SCP, is visible. The perifoveal arcade can be visualized well at 360°.

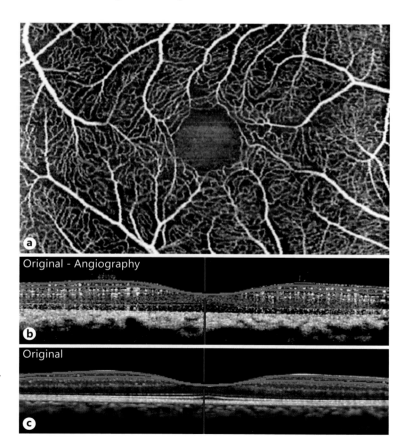

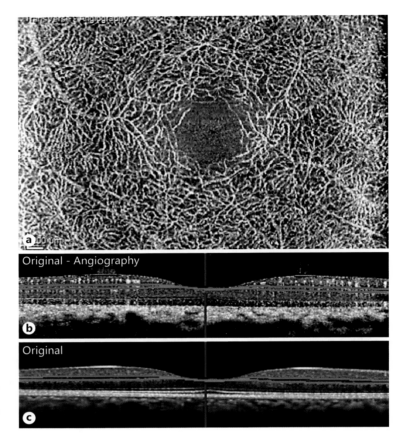

Original - Angiography

Original

Fig. 3. Visualization of the deep capillary plexus (DCP). **a** Automatically obtained OCT-A C-scan, which exactly outlines the inner nuclear layer profile (as shown in **b**, **c**). The clearly distinguishable dense capillary network surrounding the perifoveal area corresponds to the DCP. This is the first in vivo examination technique that allows fine visualization of the DCP.

This is the first in vivo examination technique that allows visualization of the DCP, which appears as a very dense, regularly anastomosed network with sinuous arborization ending in a well-distinguished draining capillary 'vortex'. Arterioles and venules are not distinctly visible. Corresponding B-scans show regularly aligned hyper-intense dots stratified in two main lines (deep and superficial), as well as an intermediate line corresponding to the interconnections between the two plexa (fig. 3a–c).

Conventional FA and OCT-A cannot be perfectly compared. This is mainly due to the bi-dimensional aspect of FA, in which all vascular structures included within the whole retina are simultaneously shown. Therefore, this type of imaging suffers some limitations due to the su-

perimposition of different layers and light scattering.

OCT-A, a depth-resolved examination technique, allows clear visualization of different structures and allows the clinician to evaluate the retinal and choroidal tissues layer-by-layer for detailed vascular analysis.

Indocyanine Green Angiography in Healthy Subjects

Indocyanine green angiography has dramatically advanced our understanding and interpretation of choroidal imaging in ophthalmology. On a normal angiogram, the choroid is difficult to define because of the numerous changes that can

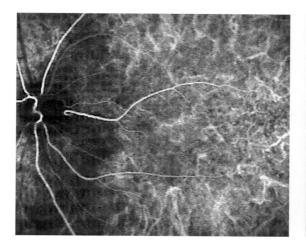

Fig. 4. Indocyanine green angiography (ICGA) during the arterial phase.

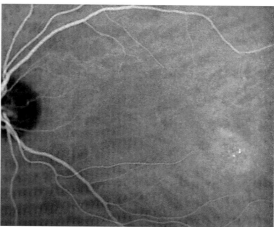

Fig. 6. ICGA during the mid-venous phase. The choroidal vessels are faintly visible.

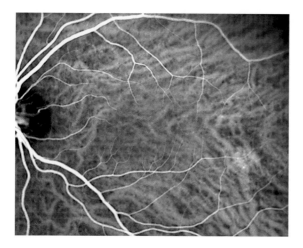

Fig. 5. ICGA during the early venous phase showing no significant changes in the large vessel choroidal network.

occur with aging or that are related to differences in pigmentation. Anatomical variants are common in the arrangement and distribution of choroidal blood vessels and in the circulatory dynamics of filling and drainage.

The dye is first seen in the choroidal arteries, which form a distinctive initial loop and an oblique pathway towards the periphery. The simultaneous filling of the cilioretinal artery can also be noted.

Arteries may emerge from different sites at variable intervals; these sites are usually perimacular and peripapillary (fig. 4). Veins show unusual pathways even more frequently, sometimes draining into the posterior pole (fig. 5, 6). However, vascular branches are usually not visible over their entire lengths due to the undulating nature of their pathways, their layered distribution and the variable calibers of vessels within the choroidal tissue; therefore, imaging them may require successive focusing.

There is a clear predominance of the venous network with difficult-to-distinguish arterial patterns. Asymmetrical arrangement of venous drainage, which is mainly directed towards the superior and inferior temporal periphery, is also evident.

Optical Coherence Tomography Angiography of the Choroid in Healthy Subjects

OCT-A, in addition providing depth-resolved information on retinal vessels, may provide further insight into choroidal flow.

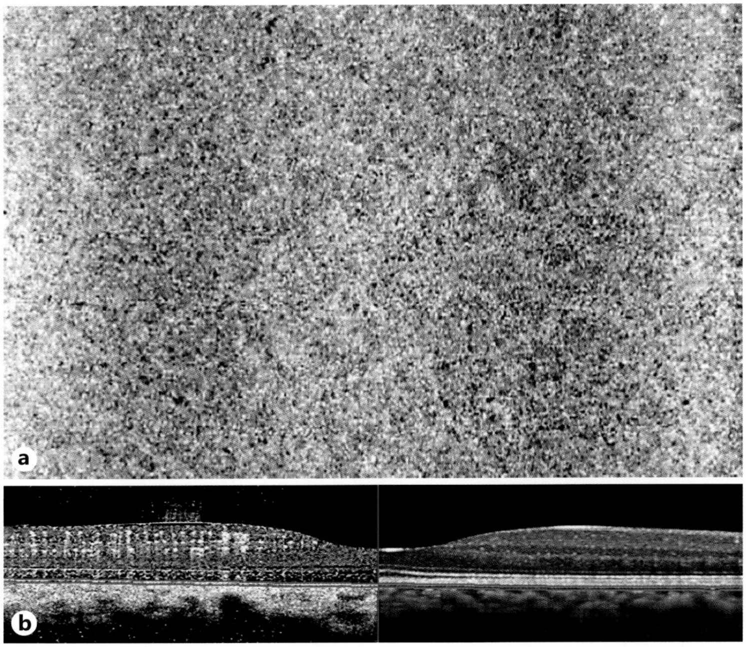

Fig. 7. Visualization of the choriocapillaris (CC). **a** A 20-μm-thick OCT-A C-scan showing the shape of Bruch's membrane (BM) profile. The C-scan was taken 10 μm below BM (as shown in **b**). Diffuse hyper-intense signal with no appreciable fine capillary network. Relatively homogenous grayish image that seems to be composed of a large number of tiny dots that are either hyper- or hypo-intense. This pattern could correspond to the very richly anastomosed vascular layer of the CC.

Choriocapillaris

The information gained by segmenting different levels that are deeper than Bruch's membrane is still limited and not fully understood. Starting from Bruch's membrane, for a 20-μm-distance toward the choroidal-scleral interface, different C-scans of Bruch's membrane profile show a relatively homogenous grayish aspect.

This aspect seems composed by a large number of tiny dots that either hyper- or hypo-intense; a few of them are moderately bigger.

This homogenous pattern could correspond to the very richly anastomosed vascular layer of the choriocapillaris. No vascular channels are clearly detectable at this level (fig. 7a, b).

Choroid (Sattler's Layer)

Different C-scans of 30-μm-thickness each taken deeper than choriocapillaris allow the analysis of the so-called Sattler's layer (a medium choroidal vessel layer). This layer is clearly visible on B-scans with a quite continuous hyper-intense signal mixed with some hypo-intense structures.

The corresponding C-scan shows many hypo-intense, linear (black, tubular) entities resembling the medium vessel network in an almost continuous hyper-intense grayish background (fig. 8a, b).

The reason we are unable to distinguish a fine, hyper-intense vascular network is because of the attenuation of signal induced by the structures above. This phenomenon is mainly due to the reflective properties of the retinal pigment epithelium and the diffusion of the hyper-intense and homogeneous signal coming from the choriocapillaris.

Choroid (Haller's Layer)

Deeper again, C-scan segmentation allows the visualization of large choroidal vessels (the so-called Haller's layer). B-scan sections show alternative areas of hypo- (black, tubular) and hyper-intense (greyish, diffuse) signal corresponding to

Coscas · Lupidi · Coscas

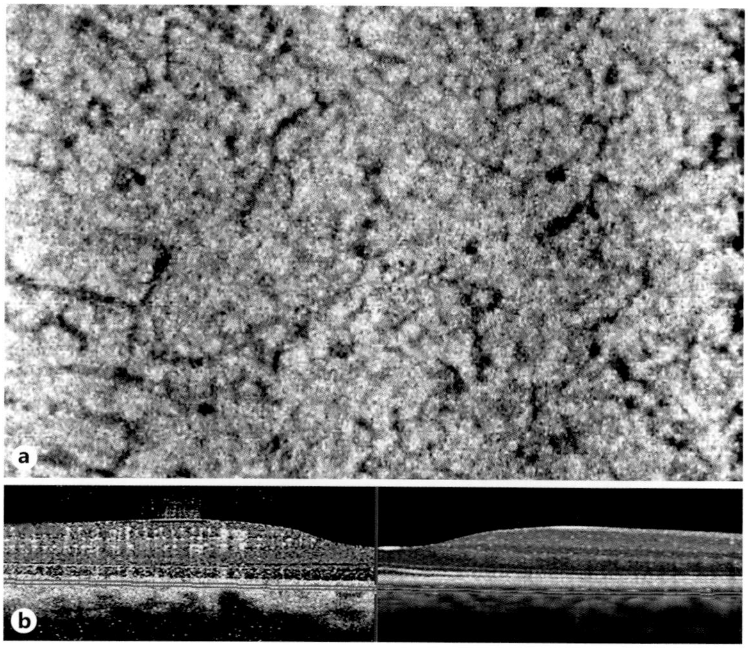

Fig. 8. Sattler's layer (medium choroidal vessels). **a** A 20-µm-thick OCT-A C-scan showing the shape of BM profile. The C-scan was taken 70 µm below BM (as shown in **b**). The diffuse hyper-intense signal due to the CC does not allow clear visualization of the medium choroidal vessels. Several hypo-intense (black) linear structures on a greyish background, probably representing the choroidal vessels present at this level, are appreciable in this C-scan section; they are partially masked by the hyper-intense signal diffusing from the CC.

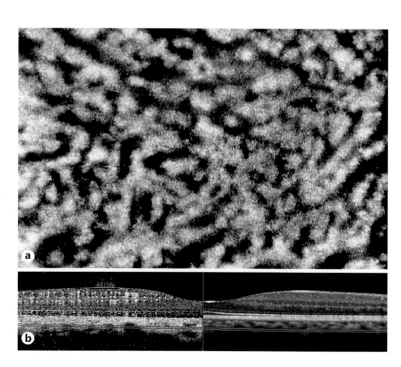

Fig. 9. Haller's layer (large choroidal vessels). **a** A 20-µm OCT-A C-scan showing the shape of BM profile. The C-scan was taken 140 µm below BM (as shown in **b**). Numerous hypo-intense linear structures (black, tubular) are evident on a greyish background. These are related to the presence of large choroidal vessels at this level. As for Sattler's layer, the decorrelation signal coming from these vessels is masked by the influence of the structures above (mainly the CC but also Sattler's layer).

these vessels, which are of much larger caliber than those in Sattler's layer (fig. 9a, b). C-scans show that the signal in this layer is discontinuous with multiple interruptions.

Even in this case, this aspect is caused by signal attenuation due to the structures above (mainly the choriocapillaris but also Sattler's layer).

References

1 Sulzbacher F, Kiss C, Munk M, et al: Diagnostic evaluation of type 2 (classic) choroidal neovascularization: optical coherence tomography, indocyanine green angiography, an fluorescein angiography. Am J Ophthalmol 2011;152: 799–806.e1.

2 Snodderly DM, Weinhaus RS, Choi JC: Neural-vascular relationships in central retina of macaque monkeys (Macacafascicularis). J Neurosci 1992;12:1169–1193.

3 Weinhaus RS, Burke JM, Delori FC, et al: Comparison of fluorescein angiography with microvascular anatomy of macaque retina. Exp Eye Res 1995;61:1–16.

4 Mendis KR, Balaratnasingam C, Yu P, et al: Correlation of histologic and clinical images to determine the diagnostic value of fluorescein angiography for studying capillary detail. Invest Ophthalmol Vis Sci 2010;51:5864–5859.

5 Spaide RF, Klancnik JM Jr, Cooney MJ: Retinal vascular layers imaged by fluorescein angiography and optical coherence tomography angiography. JAMA Ophthalmol 2015;133:45–50.

6 Moult E, Choi W, Waheed NK, et al: Ultrahigh-speed swept-source OCT angiography in exudative AMD. Ophthalmic Surg Lasers Imaging Retina 2014; 45:496–505.

7 Jia Y, Bailey ST, Wilson DJ, et al: Quantitative optical coherence tomography angiography of choroidal neovascularization in age-related macular degeneration. Ophthalmology 2014;121:1435–1444.

8 Yannuzzi LA, Rohrer KT, Tindel LJ, et al: Fluorescein angiography complication survey. Ophthalmology 1986;93: 611–617.

9 Laser Institute of America: American National Standard for Safe Use of Lasers, ANSI Z136. Orlando, FL, Laser Institute of America, 2007.

10 Bonnin S, Mané V, Couturier A, et al: New insight into the macular deep vascular plexus imaged by optical coherence tomography angiography. Retina 2015;35:2347–2352.

Prof. Gabriel Coscas
Centre Hospitalier Intercommunal de Créteil
40 Avenue de Verdun
FR–94000 Créteil (France)
E-Mail gabriel.coscas@gmail.com

Bandello F, Souied EH, Querques G (eds): OCT Angiography in Retinal and Macular Diseases.
Dev Ophthalmol. Basel, Karger, 2016, vol 56, pp 45–51 (DOI: 10.1159/000442776)

Optical Coherence Tomography Angiography of Type 1 Neovascularization in Age-Related Macular Degeneration

Nicholas A. Iafe[a] · Nopasak Phasukkijwatana[a] · David Sarraf[a, b]

[a]Stein Eye Institute, David Geffen School of Medicine at University of California Los Angeles, and [b]Greater Los Angeles VA Healthcare Center, Los Angeles, Calif., USA

Abstract

Age-related macular degeneration continues to be the leading cause of severe central vision loss in older adults of European descent. Optical coherence tomography angiography (OCT-A) enables more accurate identification of type 1 neovascularization in age-related macular degeneration than traditional fluorescein and indocyanine green angiographies. In addition, OCT-A facilitates the morphological classification of type 1 lesions, including features characteristic of early, mature, and fibrotic lesions. Vessel complex analysis, including lesion area and capillary density quantification, can also be readily measured and monitored over time. Performing this analysis following anti-vascular endothelial growth factor therapy may lead to a better understanding of the efficacies and responses to such treatments. Although some limitations currently exist, OCT-A is a promising imaging modality that could prove to have profound implications if incorporated into regular clinical practice.

© 2016 S. Karger AG, Basel

Age-related macular degeneration (AMD) continues to be the leading cause of blindness among individuals older than 50 years of age in the developed world [1]. Neovascular AMD is the etiology for severe vision loss in 90% of AMD cases. Three lesion subtypes, best classified on the basis of spectral domain optical coherence tomography (OCT), comprise the neovascular form of this disease [2]. Type 1 neovascularization originates from the choriocapillaris and is localized under the retinal pigment epithelium. Type 2 neovascularization also originates from the choriocapillaris but extends through the retinal pigment epithelium and is localized in the subretinal compartment. Type 3 neovascularization originates from the deep retinal capillary plexus [2–4] and is located in the outer retina. Type 1 neovascularization is the most common neovascular subtype of AMD [5].

Recent advancements in OCT angiography (OCT-A) have provided retinologists with a window to directly identify the morphologies of neovascular subtypes in AMD. OCT-A enables more accurate identification of type 1 lesions compared to traditional fluorescein angiography (FA). While FA can identify the superficial retinal capillary plexus, this imaging modality poorly visualizes the deep retinal capillary plexus and the choroid. Pigment epithelial detachment (PED) may demonstrate pooling or stippled fluorescence with FA, but the identification of the causative neovascular complex is very challenging and only minimally improved with indocyanine green angiography. Conversely, OCT-A utilizes amplitude or phase decorrelation technology with high-frequency and dense volumetric scanning to detect red blood cell movement and to visualize blood vessels at various depth-resolved levels of the retina and choroid [3]. As opposed to FA and indocyanine green angiography, in which the presence of an occult choroidal neovascular membrane is inferred by the presence of pooling within a PED and/or the identification of a hot spot, OCT-A reveals the vessels themselves and enables one to more accurately identify and evaluate the morphology of the neovascular complex.

OCT-A of type 1 neovascularization has lead to a detailed assessment of the microvascular morphologies of these vessel complexes, which are typically hidden under a PED. Numerous studies have identified the different morphologies of these neovascular lesions and have applied varying descriptive terms to label these structures, which are best visualized with OCT-A. These labels include 'umbrella vessels', 'seafan and medusa vessels', 'tangled network pattern', and 'pruned vascular and blossoming tree' [3, 6, 7]. This complicated and indistinct nomenclature has caused confusion in the retina community, and a simpler classification system will certainly evolve that may reflect the chronicity of type 1 neovascularization as identified with OCT-A.

Though the precise precipitating stimulus for angiogenesis in AMD remains to be elucidated, the development of neovascular complexes has been shown to be highly dependent on the presence of vascular endothelial growth factor (VEGF) [8–10]. Hypoperfusion or alteration of the choriocapillaris is often noted in OCT-A in association with type 1 complexes [3, 11–13] and is likely one cause of localized increases in VEGF production. The newly established VEGF gradient stimulates the propagation of vascular endothelial cells to form new capillaries [8]. When imaged with OCT-A in this early or acute phase, the neovascularization has the appearance of a tangled web of fine vessels (fig. 1) [8, 14]. Muakkassa et al. [14] performed OCT-A on treatment-naïve eyes with type 1 neovascularization, and the lesions were typically small (less than 1 mm^2) and comprised of a round tuft of small-caliber capillaries without dilated core feeder vessels.

Chronic type 1 lesions have been noted to demonstrate a distinctly different morphology. In the largest study to date using OCT-A to describe chronic type 1 lesions previously treated with multiple intravitreal anti-VEGF injections, Kuehlewein and associates [3] analyzed 33 eyes with AMD and PED associated with type 1 lesions that were large and mature; these averaged 5.79 mm^2 in area. Of note, 75% of the cases showed a highly organized vascular complex with vessels branching from a core trunk (fig. 2) and multiple large, dilated feeder vessels (fig. 3). The existence of well-perfused feeder vessels in chronically treated type 1 lesions has also been identified by Coscas and associates [15]. It has been hypothesized that the feeder vessels and central trunk are more resistant to anti-VEGF therapy because their endothelial cells are protected by overlying pericytes, whereas the finer branching vessels contain unprotected endothelial cells, rendering them more responsive to continued anti-VEGF therapy [16, 17]. In his seminal paper, Spaide [8] highlights the distinction between angiogenesis and arterio-

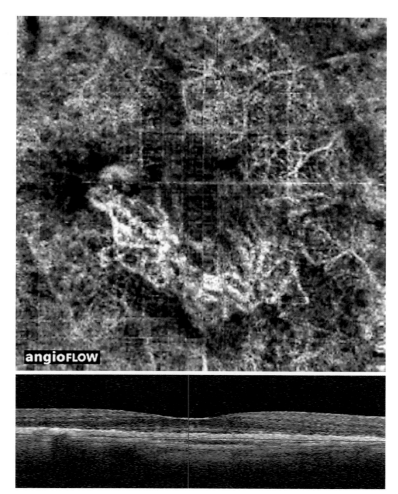

Fig. 1. An 86-year-old patient with treatment-naïve type 1 neovascularization in the right eye. (Top) A 3 mm × 3 mm motion-corrected optical coherence tomography (OCT) angiogram imaged on Avanti RTVue OCTA device showing well-circumscribed choroidal neovascularization with a tangled web of vessels. A quilting artifact due to motion is present. (Bottom) Corresponding spectral domain OCT B-scan with segmentation lines. The authors would like to acknowledge and credit Dr. Nadia Waheed and Dr. Emily Cole for providing these images.

genesis and proposes a theory of vascular abnormalization to describe the altered morphology of chronically treated type 1 neovascular complexes. Spaide theorizes that the process of closing smaller pericyte-poor vessels within a neovascular complex in response to anti-VEGF leads to increased vascular resistance within the lesion. The remaining pericyte-rich vessels subsequently experience higher flow and higher intraluminal pressure, thereby creating a stimulus for arteriogenesis and increased vessel size. A cycle of regrowth and pruning of the immature, pericyte-

poor vessels at the leading edge of the type 1 complex takes place in response to anti-VEGF therapy, while the mature, dilated pericyte-rich core vessels progressively enlarge. This cycling has been shown to carry a risk of evolution toward subretinal fibrosis [18, 19].

OCT-A has also been employed to study the late fibrotic stage of type 1 neovascularization in AMD. Miere and associates [7] analyzed 49 eyes diagnosed with subretinal fibrosis complicating neovascular AMD, 39 of which were either type 1 or combined type 1 and type 2 lesions. OCT-A

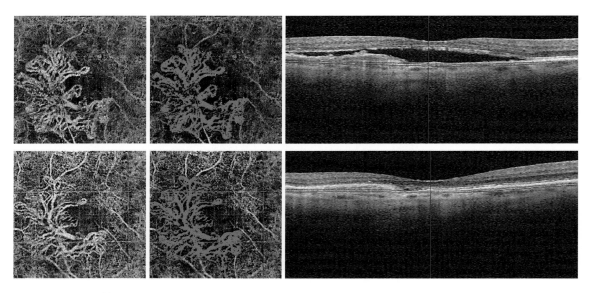

Fig. 2. A 77-year-old male patient with type 1 neovascularization in the right eye, with a visual acuity of 20/40. The patient's status following 6 aflibercept injections and 7 ranibizumab injections is shown. (Top left) 3 mm x 3 mm OCT angiography (OCT-A) en face projection image of a mature type 1 complex with large feeder vessels and multiple dilated core vessels identified. (Top middle) Corresponding color-coded vessel complex for density analysis. (Top right) OCT B-scan image showing slab segmentation through the pigment epithelial detachment. (Bottom row) Follow-up OCT-A 8 weeks later (interim treatment: 2 aflibercept injections). (Bottom left) 3 mm x 3 mm OCT-A en face projection image of the type 1 complex. (Bottom middle) Corresponding color-coded complex for vessel density analysis. (Bottom right) OCT B-scan image showing slab segmentation. Note that the many large, dilated vessels of this mature type 1 complex are unaffected by additional anti-vascular endothelial growth factor therapy, although the finer vascular plexus may show some attenuation. The lesion area was 3.08 mm² at baseline and 3.08 mm² at follow-up; the vessel density was 47% at baseline and 43% at follow-up.

demonstrated blood flow related to a persistent neovascular complex within the fibrotic scar in 46 of the 49 eyes [7]. Analysis of these complexes revealed large, dilated vessels with or without vascular loops and interlacing networks, but they typically consisted of only large, mature vessels without an associated fine dense capillary plexus. Most fibrotic lesions also had large flow void areas of the choriocapillaris or dark halos.

Additionally, OCT-A has been utilized to characterize the response of type 1 neovascularization to antiangiogenic therapy. Muakkassa and associates [14] studied six patients with treatment-naïve choroidal neovascularization (CNV),

four of which had type 1 lesions. Eyes were scanned before anti-VEGF treatment and at follow-up visits in order to assess the area of each neovascular lesion and its greatest linear dimension (GLD). Follow-up images taken 2–9.5 weeks after initial injection revealed a 29.8% average decrease in CNV area and a 23.6% decrease in its GLD [14]. All patients also experienced improvement or stabilization of their best-corrected visual acuity. Muakkassa et al. [14] suggested that quantitative OCT-A may be useful in determining treatment response and may allow for early detection of inadequately treated lesions.

Kuehlewein and associates [3] investigated interval changes in lesion area and vessel density in

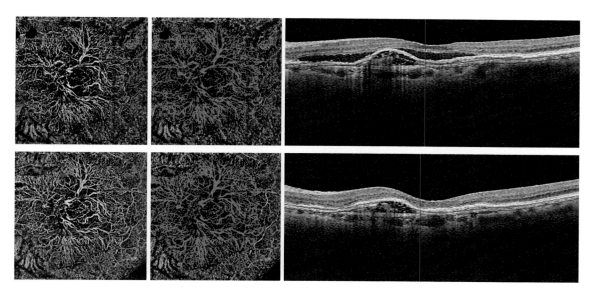

Fig. 3. A 93-year-old female patient with type 1 neovascularization in the left eye, with a visual acuity of 20/60. The patient's status following 1 aflibercept injection and 16 ranibizumab injections is shown. (Top left) 6 mm x 6 mm OCT-A en face projection image of the mature type 1 complex shows many large, dilated vessels radiating from the center and several large core feeder vessels. (Top middle) Corresponding color-coded vessel complex for density analysis. (Top right) OCT B-scan image showing slab segmentation through the vascularized pigment epithelium detachment. (Bottom row) Follow-up OCT-A 12 weeks later (interim treatment: 1 aflibercept injection). (Bottom left) 6 mm x 6 mm OCT-A en face projection image of the neovascular complex. (Bottom middle) Corresponding color-coded complex for vessel density analysis. (Bottom right) OCT B-scan image showing slab segmentation. Note that the large dilated vessels and the core trunk of this mature type 1 complex are unaffected by additional anti-vascular endothelial growth factor therapy. The lesion area was 20.52 mm^2 at baseline and 20.08 mm^2 at follow-up; the vessel density was 57% at baseline and 56% at follow-up.

chronic mature type 1 lesions in 12 patients with long-term history of anti-VEGF therapy who each received an additional injection. In this subset of patients, no statistically significant differences in lesion area or vessel density were found after the addition of interval anti-VEGF therapy (fig. 2, 3). The majority of the type 1 neovascular complexes identified in these patients contained a large central feeder vessel and multiple dilated core vessels (with pericyte-protected endothelial cells), which is indicative of the chronic mature nature of the lesions. It should be noted, however, that some smaller-caliber vessels (without pericyte-protected endothelial cells) radiating from the central trunks of some lesions did ap-

pear attenuated with the additional anti-VEGF therapy.

Despite great advancements in the identification and analysis of type 1 neovascularization with OCT-A, considerable limitations do still exist. Since split-spectrum amplitude-decorrelation technology relies on the detection of erythrocyte movement, any movement of a patient's head or eyes during image acquisition results in significant artifact production and decreased image quality [3, 7, 8, 12, 14, 15]. In addition, the generation of projection artifacts and the shadowing of the superficial capillary plexus onto the deeper layers of the retina can make it difficult to distinguish normal vessels from pathologic vessel complexes. More advanced software to remove or correct for these types of artifacts will greatly improve the utility of OCT-A in clinical practice. Furthermore, increased precision and the ability to easily modify slab segmentation for follow-up encounters is also necessary in order to more accurately evaluate changes in vessel complexes over time and following anti-VEGF therapy.

OCT-A continues to be a promising method for identifying the morphology and monitoring the treatment response of type 1 neovascularization and PED, as conventional angiography cannot adequately visualize occult pathologic vessels [20]. The ability to identify neovascular complexes and their distinct microvascular structures via OCT-A empowers the retinologist to directly gauge and measure the response of pathologic vessels to intravitreal anti-VEGF therapy or other novel therapeutic agents. Qualitative assessment of morphological changes in a vessel complex in response to therapy may be valuable. Important quantitative measurements include baseline and follow-up lesion area, lesion vessel density, and GLD. This type of qualitative and quantitative OCT-A analysis performed on a larger scale may be used to better assess the efficacy of anti-VEGF treatment in research trials, leading to more efficacious pharmacotherapeutics, and in the clinical arena, leading to more optimal care for patients with neovascular AMD.

References

1 Eye Diseases Prevalence Research Group: Causes and prevalence of visual impairment among adults in the United States. Arch Ophthalmol 2004;122:477–485.

2 Freund KB, Zweifel SA, Engelbert M: Do we need a new classification for choroidal neovascularization in age-related macular degeneration? Retina 2010;30:1333–1349.

3 Kuehlewein L, Bansal M, Lenis TL, Iafe NA, Sadda SR, Bonini Filho MA, De Carlo TE, Waheed NK, Duker JS, Sarraf D: Optical coherence tomography angiography of type 1 neovascularization in age-related macular degeneration. Am J Ophthalmol 2015;160:739–748.e2.

4 Nagiel A, Sarraf D, Sadda SR, Spaide RF, Jung JJ, Bhavsar KV, Ameri H, Querques G, Freund KB: Type 3 neovascularization: evolution, association with pigment epithelial detachment, and treatment response as revealed by spectral domain optical coherence tomography. Retina (Philadelphia, Pa.) 2015;35:638–647.

5 Jung JJ, Chen CY, Mrejen S, Gallego-Pinazo R, Xu L, Marsiglia M, Boddu S, Freund KB: The incidence of neovascular subtypes in newly diagnosed neovascular age-related macular degeneration. Am J Ophthalmol 2014;158:769–779.e2.

6 Kawamura A, Yuzawa M, Mori R, Haruyama M, Tanaka K: Indocyanine green angiographic and optical coherence tomographic findings support classification of polypoidal choroidal vasculopathy into two types. Acta Ophthalmol 2013;91:e474–e481.

7 Miere A, Semoun O, Cohen SY, El Ameen A, Srour M, Jung C, Oubraham H, Querques G, Souied EH: Optical coherence tomography angiography features of subretinal fibrosis in age-related macular degeneration. Retina (Philadelphia, Pa.) 2015;35:2275–2284.

8 Spaide RF: Optical coherence tomography angiography signs of vascular abnormalization with antiangiogenic therapy for choroidal neovascularization. Am J Ophthalmol 2015;160:6–16.

9 Adams RH, Alitalo K: Molecular regulation of angiogenesis and lymphangiogenesis. Nat Rev Mol Cell Biol 2007;8:464–478.

10 Weis SM, Cheresh DA: Tumor angiogenesis: molecular pathways and therapeutic targets. Nat Med 2011;17:1359–1370.

11 Jia Y, Bailey ST, Wilson DJ, Tan O, Klein ML, Flaxel CJ, Potsaid B, Liu JJ, Lu CD, Kraus MF, Fujimoto JG, Huang D: Quantitative optical coherence tomography angiography of choroidal neovascularization in age-related macular degeneration. Ophthalmology 2014;121:1435–1444.

12 Moult E, Choi W, Waheed NK, Adhi M, Lee B, Lu CD, Jayaraman V, Potsaid B, Rosenfeld PJ, Duker JS, Fujimoto JG: Ultrahigh-speed sweptsource OCT angiography in exudative AMD. Ophthalmic Surg Lasers Imaging Retina 2014;45:496–505.

13 Grossniklaus HE, Green WR: Choroidal neovascularization. Am J Ophthalmol 2004;137:496–503.

14 Muakkassa NW, Chin AT, de Carlo T, Klein KA, Baumal CR, Witkin AJ, Duker JS, Waheed NK: Characterizing the effect of anti-vascular endothelial growth factor therapy on treatment-naive choroidal neovascularization using optical coherence tomography angiography. Retina (Philadelphia, Pa.) 2015;35:2252–2259.

15 Coscas G, Lupidi M, Coscas F, Français C, Cagini C, Souied EH: Optical coherence tomography angiography during follow-up: qualitative and quantitative analysis of mixed type I and II choroidal neovascularization after vascular endothelial growth factor trap therapy. Ophthalmic Res 2015;54:57–63.

16 Bellou S, Pentheroudakis G, Murphy C, Fotsis T: Anti-angiogenesis in cancer therapy: Hercules and hydra. Cancer Lett 2013;338:219–228.

17 Benjamin LE, Hemo I, Keshet E: A plasticity window for blood vessel remodeling is defined by pericyte coverage of the preformed endothelial network and is regulated by PDGF-B and VEGF. Development 1998;125:1591–1598.

18 Bloch SB, Lund-Andersen H, Sander B, Larsen M: Subfoveal fibrosis in eyes with neovascular age-related macular degeneration treated with intravitreal ranibizumab. Am J Ophthalmol 2013; 156:116–124.

19 Channa R, Sophie R, Bagheri S, Shah SM, Wang J, Adeyemo O, Sodhi A, Wenick A, Ying HS, Campochiaro PA: Regression of choroidal neovascularization results in macular atrophy in anti-vascular endothelial growth factor-treated eyes. Am J Ophthalmol 2015;159: 9–19.

20 Peden MC, Suñer IJ, Hammer ME, Grizzard WS: Long-term outcomes in eyes receiving fixed-interval dosing of anti-vascular endothelial growth factor agents for wet age related macular degeneration. Ophthalmology 2015;122: 803–809.

David Sarraf, MD
Retinal Disorders and Ophthalmic Genetics Division, Stein Eye Institute
David Geffen School of Medicine at UCLA, 100 Stein Plaza
Los Angeles, CA 90095 (USA)
E-Mail dsarraf@ucla.edu

Bandello F, Souied EH, Querques G (eds): OCT Angiography in Retinal and Macular Diseases.
Dev Ophthalmol. Basel, Karger, 2016, vol 56, pp 52–56 (DOI: 10.1159/000442777)

Optical Coherence Tomography Angiography of Type 2 Neovascularization in Age-Related Macular Degeneration

Eric H. Souied[a] · Ala El Ameen[a] · Oudy Semoun[a] · Alexandra Miere[a] · Giuseppe Querques[a, b] · Salomon Yves Cohen[a]

[a]Department of Ophthalmology, Centre Hospitalier Intercommunal de Créteil, Paris Est University, Créteil, France;
[b]Department of Ophthalmology IRCCS San Raffaele Scientific Institute University Vita-Salute San Raffaele, Milan, Italy

Abstract

Well-defined choroidal neovascularization, known as type 2 neovascularization (NV) or classic NV, is the least representative phenotype of exudative age-related macular degeneration. Clinical aspects of type 2 NV have been widely described in the literature, and to date fluorescein angiography remains the gold standard for imaging age-related macular degeneration at initial presentation. Optical coherence tomography angiography (OCT-A) can be used to image vessels based on flow characteristics without any dye injection. Type 2 NV can be visualized using OCT-A with very typical patterns. A neovascular membrane appears as either a medusa-shaped complex or a glomerulus-shaped lesion in the outer retina and the choriocapillaris layer. Furthermore, in the choriocapillaris layer, the external borders of the lesion appear as a dark ring in most cases, and one or more central feeder vessels that extend deeply into the more profound choroidal layers are visible. Identification of type 2 NV is easily feasible for any clinician using OCT-A, especially in areas where there are normally no vessels, like in subretinal space, if the interpretation rules are respected.

© 2016 S. Karger AG, Basel

Age-related macular degeneration (AMD) is the leading cause of blindness after 50 years in age in the Western world [1]. AMD is a phenotypically heterogeneous disease, including atrophic (dry) and exudative (wet) forms. More than 80% of severe visual loss cases in AMD arise from choroidal neovascularization (CNV) and its consequences: exudation, bleeding and disciform scar [2]. The exudative form is characterized by abnormal growth of newly formed vessels within the macula. Gass [3] used enucleated eyes and classified neovascular growth patterns as subretinal pigment epithelial (type 1, or 'occults' CNV), preretinal pigment epithelial (type 2), or combined. Well-defined CNV, or type 2 neovascularization (NV), also called classic CNV or preepithelial CNV, is the least representative phenotype of exudative AMD, accounting for 17.6% of all neovascular AMD cases [4].

Clinical aspects of type 2 NV have been widely described in the literature. To date, fluorescein angiography remains the gold standard for

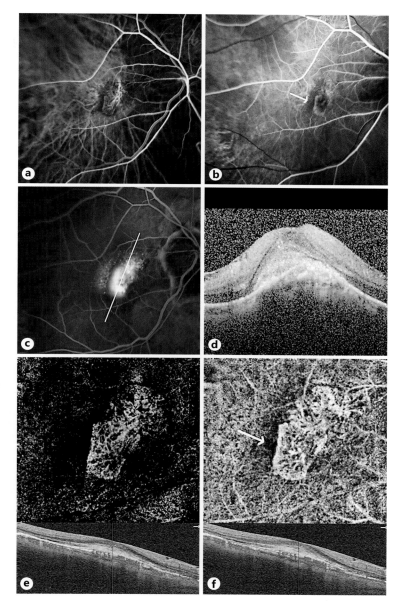

Fig. 1. Multimodal imaging of the right eye of a 79-year-old woman showing type 2 neovascularization (NV) naïve to treatment. **a** Early phase of indocyanine green angiography; **b**, **c** early (**b**) and late (**c**) phases of fluorescein angiography (FA); **d** Spectral domain optical coherence tomography (OCT) through the white dotted line. *En face* OCT angiography segments of the outer retina (**e**) of a hyperflow medusa-shaped lesion that was also visible when segmentation was performed at the level of the choriocapillaris layer (**f**). The white arrow shows the dark ring in the early phase of FA and around the medusa-shaped lesion observed in the choriocapillaris layer.

imaging AMD at initial presentation if neovascular complications are anticipated. Type 2 NV presents a well-demarcated area of hyperfluorescence (corresponding to the neovascular membrane) in the early frames of an angiogram. Late phases are marked by a progressive leakage of dye from this area [5].

Type 2 NV can be visualized using optical coherence tomography angiography (OCT-A) with very typical patterns. The neovascular membrane appears either as a medusa-shaped complex (fig. 1) or a glomerulus-shaped lesion (fig. 2) in the outer retina [6]. The medusa-shaped complex is characterized by a well-

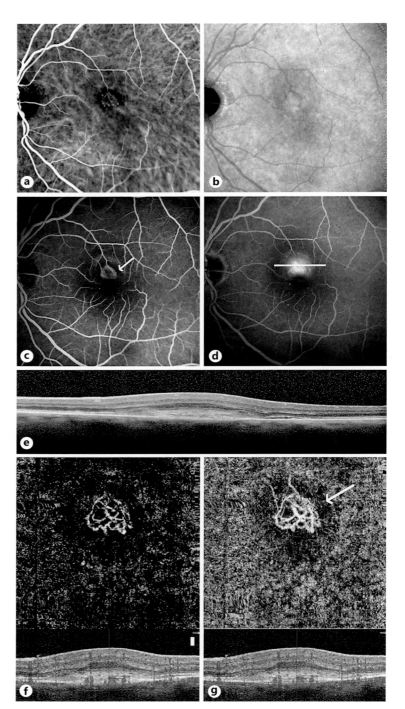

Fig. 2. Multimodal imaging of the right eye of an 86-year-old man showing type 2 NV naïve to treatment. **a, b** Early (**a**) and late (**b**) phases of indocyanine green angiography; **c, d** early (**c**) and late (**d**) phases of FA show typical classic NV. **e** Spectral domain OCT through the hyperfluorescent lesion shows a hyperreflective preretinal lesion (type 2 NV). *En face* OCT angiography segments of the outer retina (**f**) and choriocapillaris layer (**g**) of the hyperflow glomerulus-shaped lesion. The white arrow shows the dark ring in the early phase of FA and around the glomerulus-shaped lesion in the choriocapillaris layer.

defined oval shape, generally formed by a very dense high-flow network at diagnosis because of the high activity of this kind of choroidal new vessel. The glomerulus-shaped lesion is usually rounded, well defined, and full of a very dense maze of small new vessels. Anatomically, the retina is supplied by 2 capillary plexa: the superficial capillary plexus and the deep capillary plexus. The superficial capillary plexus is located between the internal limiting membrane and the posterior part of the inner plexiform layer, while the deep plexus is situated in the inner nuclear layer [7]. No vascular abnormality is detected in either the superficial or deep retinal capillary layers. Two automatic segmentations on OCT-A are interesting for type 2 NV secondary to AMD. The first, called the 'outer retina', is delimited between the inner nuclear layer and Bruch's membrane (BM), and the second, called the 'choriocapillaris layer' is located under BM. At the pathophysiologic level, type 2 NV involves choroidal new vessels that cross BM and grow up above the neurosensory retina. This feature allows us to visualize these lesions on the outer retina. A glomerulus- or medusa-shaped lesion can also be observed on segmentations performed at the level of the choriocapillaris. Furthermore, in the choriocapillaris layer, the external borders of the lesion appear as a dark ring in most cases [6] (fig. 1, 2). One or more central feeder vessels that expand in radial branches and continue deeply into the more profound choroidal layers are visible. In a short series, the feeder vessel was identified in 9 cases out of 14 [6]. It is exceptional to distinguish and recognize the afferent of the efferent branches.

The complex morphology of type 2 NV changes after treatment using vascular endothelial growth factor antagonists, leading to a decrease in size and density, and the prominent tangle becomes less compact. After long-term treatment, the neovascular lesion becomes fibrotic and its appearance on OCT-A changes [8].

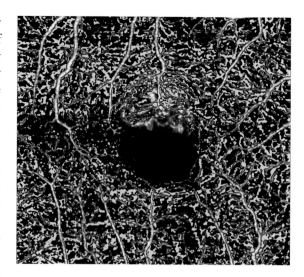

Fig. 3. Colorization of retinal vascularization and type 2 NV in the right eye of an 86-year-old man. The superficial plexus is shown in blue, the deep capillary plexus is shown in yellow, and the type 2 NV is show in red.

OCT-A is a novel and noninvasive imaging tool that allows visualization of retinal microvasculature by detecting intravascular blood flow based on split spectrum amplitude decorrelation angiography [6–11] without any dye injection.

Analysis of OCT-A images may be subjected to many artifacts, like projection artifacts, which can lead to misinterpretation, and the detection of such artifacts requires a clinician to perform an interactive evaluation [12]. Conversely, this new technology allows such great resolution of vascular layers that we can colorize each one and overlap them (fig. 3).

By definition, type 2 NV is preepithelial, so any vessel in this area ('outer retina') can be considered type 2 NV and abnormal.

Identification of type 2 NV appears easily feasible for any clinician using OCT-A, especially in areas where there are normally no vessels, like in the subretinal space, if the interpretation rules are respected [12].

References

1 Friedman DS, O'Colmain BJ, Munoz B, et al: Prevalence of age- related macular degeneration in the United States. Arch Ophthalmol 2004;122:564–572.

2 Ferris FL 3rd, Fine SL, Hyman L: Age-related macular degeneration and blindness due to neovascular maculopathy. Arch Ophthalmol 1984;102:1640–1642.

3 Gass JD: Biomicroscopic and histopathologic considerations regarding the feasibility of surgical excision of subfoveal neovascular membranes. Am J Ophthalmol 1994;118:285–298.

4 Cohen SY, Creuzot-Garcher C, Darmon J, et al: Types of choroidal neovascularization in newly diagnosed exudative age-related macular degeneration. Br J Ophthalmol 2007;91:1173–1176.

5 Lopez PF, Lambert HM, Grossniklaus HE, et al: Well-defined subfoveal choroidal neovascular membranes in age-related macular degeneration. Ophthalmology 1993;100:415–422.

6 El Ameen A, Cohen SY, Semoun O, et al: Type 2 neovascularization secondary to age-related macular degeneration imaged by optical coherence tomography angiography. Retina 2015;35:2212–2218.

7 Spaide RF, Klancnik JM Jr, Cooney MJ: Retinal vascular layers imaged by fluorescein angiography and optical coherence tomography angiography. JAMA Ophthalmol 2015;133:45–50.

8 Miere A, Semoun O, Cohen SY, et al: Optical coherence tomography angiography features of subretinal fibrosis in age-related macular. Retina 2015;35:2275–2284.

9 Kuehlewein L, Dansingani KK, de Carlo TE, et al: Optical coherence tomography angiography of type 3 neovascularization secondary to age-related macular degeneration. Retina 2015;35:2229–2235.

10 Kuehlewein L, Bansal M, Lenis TL, et al: Optical coherence tomography angiography of type 1 neovascularization in age-related macular degeneration. Am J Ophthalmol 2015;160:739–748.e2.

11 Jia Y, Tan O, Tokayer J, et al: Split-spectrum amplitude-decorrelation angiography with optical coherence tomography. Opt Express 2012;20:4710–4725.

12 Spaide RF, Fujimoto JG, Waheed NK: Image artifacts in optical coherence tomography angiography. Retina 2015;35:2163–2180.

Eric H. Souied
Department of Ophthalmology
Centre Hospitalier Intercommunal de Créteil
Universite Paris Est Créteil
40 Avenue de Verdun
FR–94000 Créteil (France)
E-Mail eric.souied@chicreteil.fr

Bandello F, Souied EH, Querques G (eds): OCT Angiography in Retinal and Macular Diseases.
Dev Ophthalmol. Basel, Karger, 2016, vol 56, pp 57–61 (DOI: 10.1159/000442779)

Optical Coherence Tomography Angiography Features of Type 3 Neovascularization in Age-Related Macular Degeneration

Giuseppe Querques[a, b] · Alexandra Miere[a] · Eric H. Souied[a]

[a]Department of Ophthalmology, Centre Hospitalier Intercommunal de Créteil, Paris Est University, Créteil, France;
[b]Department of Ophthalmology IRCCS San Raffaele Scientific Institute University Vita-Salute San Raffaele, Milan, Italy

Abstract

Purpose: To characterize the imaging features of type 3 neovascularization secondary to exudative age-related macular degeneration on optical coherence tomography (OCT) angiography (OCTA). **Methods:** Patients diagnosed with treatment-naïve early-stage type 3 neovascularization underwent multimodal imaging, including color retinal photography or multicolor imaging, fluorescein angiography, indocyanine green angiography, spectral-domain OCT and OCTA. The OCTA features of type 3 neovascularization were analyzed and correlated with the findings on angiography and spectral-domain OCT. **Results:** OCTA showed lesions characterized by a retinal-retinal anastomosis. These lesions emerged from the deep capillary plexus and formed a clear, tuft-shaped, high-flow network in the outer retinal segment in all eyes, abutting in the subretinal pigment epithelium space. In most cases, a small, clew-like lesion was present in the choriocapillaris segment. Moreover, in some cases, this clew-like lesion seemed to be connected to the choroid through a small-caliber vessel. **Conclusion:** OCTA of treatment-naïve type 3 neovascularization shows high-flow, tuft-shaped, abnormal outer retinal proliferation that is almost consistently associated with a small, clew-like lesion in the choriocapillaris layer.

© 2016 S. Karger AG, Basel

Three types of neovascularization have been described as secondary to age-related macular degeneration (AMD). According to the anatomic location of choroidal new vessels, Gass thoroughly defined type 1 and 2 choroidal neovascularization in his classical textbook of macular disease [1]. While the origin, anatomic location and imaging features and of both type 1 and 2 neovascularization are well established, type 3 neovascularization is more controversial. Introduced by

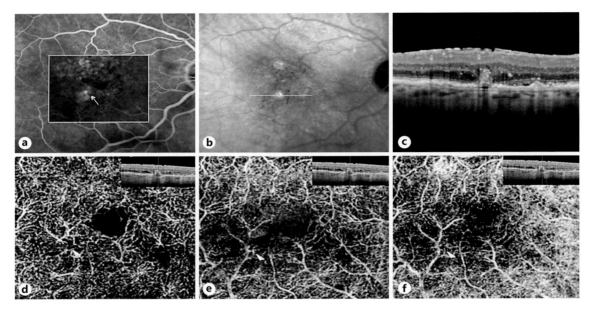

Fig. 1. Multimodal imaging of the right eye of a treatment-naïve 83-year-old male diagnosed with type 3 neovascularization. **a** Fluorescein angiography early frame demonstrates a small hyperfluorescent lesion inferior to the fovea (white arrow). **b** Late indocyanine green angiography (ICGA) frame shows a typical hot spot due to late leakage. **c** Spectral-domain optical coherence tomography (OCT) angiography (OCTA) reveals a hyper-reflective intraretinal vascular complex, emanating from the deep capillary plexus and dragging toward the subretinal pigment epithelium (RPE) space. **d–f** Three-by-three millimeter OCTA images and corresponding B-scan. The segmentation corresponding to the deep capillary plexus shows two moderately high flow, small-caliber vessels (white arrowhead in panel **d**) dragging toward the segmentation corresponding to the outer retinal layers (panel **e**), forming a tuft-shaped, high-flow lesion (white arrowhead) characterized by a retinal-retinal anastomosis, and abutting in the sub-RPE space. At the choriocapillaris level (panel **f**), there is a discrete clew-like lesion (white arrowhead).

Freund in 2008 [2], lesions described with the term type 3 neovascularization essentially encompass two previously described lesions: retinal angiomatous proliferation and chorioretinal anastomosis [3, 4]. Described by Yanuzzi as a distinct form of neovascular AMD, retinal angiomatous proliferation consists of focal neovascular proliferation from the deep retinal layer, extending into the subretinal space and possibly communicating with a choroidal neovascularization [3, 5]. Chorioretinal anastomosis, on the contrary, is defined as an intraretinal extension of type 1 neovascularization [4]. Reconciled under the term type 3 neovascularization and described as a hyperfluorescent intraretinal vascular com-

plex characterized by retinal-retinal anastomosis on conventional multimodal imaging, giving rise to a hot spot on indocyanine green angiography late frames [6], this lesion's pathophysiology remains disputable.

Optical coherence tomography angiography (OCTA) is an emerging imaging technique that allows for blood flow visualization by means of the split-spectrum amplitude-decorrelation angiography algorithm (among other technologies), thereby enabling detailed assessment of the retinal microcirculation [7]. In the particular case of type 3 neovascularization, OCTA seems particularly contributive and has revealed new information. OCTA could be a highly suitable imaging

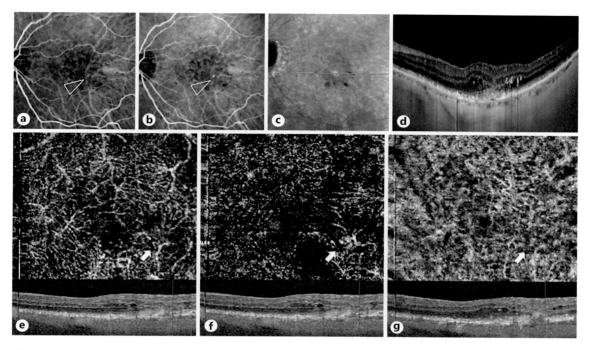

Fig. 2. Multimodal imaging of the left eye of a treatment-naïve 87-year-old female diagnosed with type 3 neovascularization. **a–c** ICGA frames demonstrate the connection between an arteriole and venule, forming a round hyperfluorescent lesion (arrowhead) temporally in the foveal avascular zone. **d** Spectral-domain OCT guided by ICGA demonstrates a hyper-reflective intraretinal complex emanating from the deep capillary plexus, apparently dragging toward the sub-RPE space, and characterized by moderate intraretinal and subretinal exudation. **e–g** Three-by-three millimeter OCTA images and corresponding B-scan. **e** OCTA deep capillary plexus segmentation, showing a high-flow third-order vessel descending toward the outer retinal layers (arrow). **f** A tuft-shaped high-flow lesion appears in the outer retinal layers, characterized by a retinal-retinal anastomosis and abutting in the sub-RPE space (arrow). **g** The choriocapillaris segmentation reveals that the tuft-shaped lesion is apparently connected to a deeper, discrete clew-like lesion.

technique for the detection, diagnosis and monitoring of these small, high-flow, peculiar intraretinal lesions.

On OCTA, type 3 neovascularization can be defined as a retinal-retinal anastomosis that emerges from the deep capillary plexus (fig. 1–4), giving rise to a high-flow, tuft-shaped neovascular lesion (fig. 1–4) in the segmentation corresponding to the outer retinal layers, finally abutting in the subretinal pigment epithelium (RPE) space. In the choriocapillaris segmentation, a small clew-like lesion corresponds to the above-mentioned tuft-shaped network (fig. 1–3). Moreover, in some cases, this glomerular lesion seems to be connected with the choroid through a small-caliber vessel (fig. 3, 4) [8].

OCTA has confirmed the hypothesis that in most cases, the early appearance of type 3 neovascularization is characterized by an intraretinal vascular complex emanating from the deep capillary plexus. This tuft-shaped intraretinal proliferation may be associated with evolving sub-RPE neovascular tissue, corresponding to a small clew-like lesion in the choriocapillaris segment. However, the presence of an early connection between the evolving sub-RPE neovascular

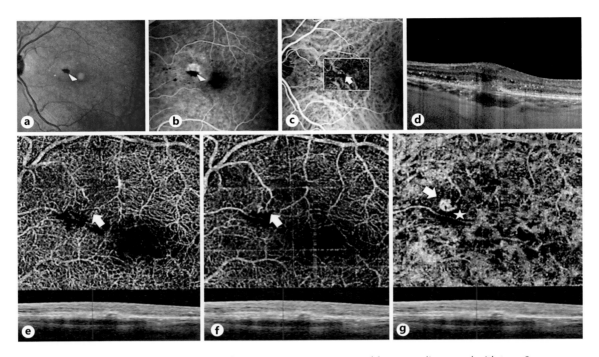

Fig. 3. Multimodal imaging of the left eye of a treatment-naïve 66-year-old woman diagnosed with type 3 neovascularization. **a** Multicolor photograph of the left eye, showing a small hemorrhage (arrowhead) superior to the fovea, as well as numerous reticular pseudodrusen. **b, c** Fluorescein angiography and ICGA show a small area of early hyperfluorescence superior to the fovea. **c** ICGA reveals a hot spot due to late leakage. No late plaque, suggesting the presence of type 1 neovascularization, was detected on ICGA. **d** Spectral-domain OCT corresponding to the hyperfluorescent area reveals a hyper-reflective intraretinal complex emanating from the deep capillary plexus and dragging toward the sub-RPE space. **e–g** Three-by-three millimeter OCTA and corresponding OCT B-scan show 2 high-flow vessels originating in the deep capillary plexus (Panel **e**, arrow, partially masked by the hemorrhage), dragging toward the outer retinal layers and descending into a tuft-shaped high-flow lesion. They are characterized by a retinal-retinal anastomosis and are abutting in the sub-RPE space (Panel **f**, arrow, partially masked by the hemorrhage). **g** The choriocapillaris segmentation reveals a deeper, small, clew-like lesion (white arrow) that seems to be connected to the choroid through a small-caliber vessel (white star).

Fig. 4. Multimodal imaging of the right eye of an 80-year-old female diagnosed with type 3 neovascularization. **a** Fluorescein angiography shows a small area of early hyperfluorescence superior to the fovea. **b** ICGA reveals a hot spot superior to the foveal avascular zone. **c** B-scan corresponding to the hyperfluorescent area demonstrates a hyper-reflective intraretinal complex emanating from the deep capillary plexus, apparently dragging toward the sub-RPE space and characterized by massive intraretinal and subretinal exudation. **d–f** Two-by-two millimeter OCTA images and corresponding B-scan. **d** OCTA deep capillary plexus segmentation discloses two vessels situated superior to the fovea and descending toward the outer retinal layers. **e** A tuft-shaped, high-flow lesion appears in the outer retinal layers, characterized by a retinal-retinal anastomosis and abutting in the sub-RPE space. **f** The choriocapillaris segmentation reveals that the tuft-shaped lesion is apparently connected to a deeper, small glomerular lesion. The glomerular lesion seemed to be connected to the choroid through a small-caliber vessel (white star). Image adapted from Miere et al. [8]. *(For figure see next page.)*

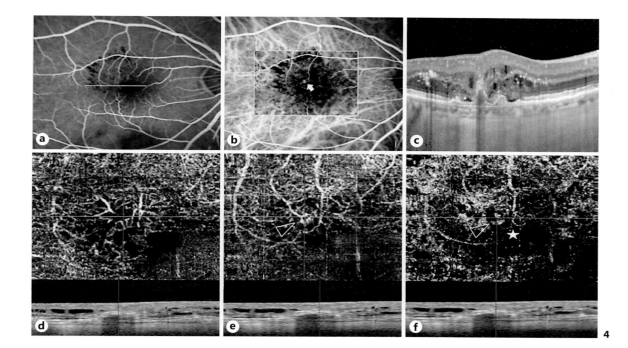

4

tissue and the choroid does not allow for the exclusion, at least in some cases of type 3 neovascularization, of a possible choroidal origin.

OCTA has confirmed to some extent the important roles of the deep capillary plexus and early evolving sub-RPE neovascularization in the formation of tuft-shaped and glomerular lesions in the pathogenesis of this particular form of neovascular AMD.

References

1 Gass JD: Stereoscopic Atlas of Macular Diseases, ed 4. St. Louis, MO, C.V. Mosby, 1997, pp 26–30.

2 Freund KB, Ho IV, Barbazetto IA, et al: Type 3 neovascularization: the expanded spectrum of retinal angiomatous proliferation. Retina 2008;28:201–211.

3 Yannuzzi LA, Negrao S, Iida T, et al: Retinal angiomatous proliferation in age-related macular degeneration. Retina 2001;21:416–434.

4 Gass JD, Agarwal A, Lavina AM, et al: Focal inner retinal hemorrhages in patients with drusen: an early sign of occult choroidal neovascularization and chorioretinal anastomosis. Retina 2003; 23:741–751.

5 Yannuzzi LA, Freund KB, Takahashi BS: Review of retinal angiomatous proliferation or type 3 neovascularization. Retina 2008;28:375–384.

6 Querques G, Souied EH, Freund KB: How has high-resolution multimodal imaging refined our understanding of the vasogenic process in type 3 neovascularization? Retina 2015;35:603–613.

7 Jia Y, Bailey ST, Wilson DJ, et al: Quantitative optical coherence tomography angiography of choroidal neovascularization in age-related macular degeneration. Ophthalmology 2014;121:1435–1444.

8 Miere A, Querques G, Semoun O, et al: Optical coherence tomography angiography in early type 3 neovascularization. Retina 2015;35:2236–2241.

Giuseppe Querques
Head – Medical Retina and Imaging Unit, Department of Ophthalmology
University Vita Salute, San Raffaele Scientific Institute
Via Olgettina, 60, IT–20132 Milan (Italy)
E-Mail querques.giuseppe@hsr.it

Bandello F, Souied EH, Querques G (eds): OCT Angiography in Retinal and Macular Diseases.
Dev Ophthalmol. Basel, Karger, 2016, vol 56, pp 62–70 (DOI: 10.1159/000442780)

Optical Coherence Tomography Angiography of Mixed Neovascularizations in Age-Related Macular Degeneration

Michelle C. Liang · Andre J. Witkin

New England Eye Center, Tufts Medical Center, Boston, Mass., USA

Abstract

Purpose: To describe the imaging of mixed neovascular age-related macular degeneration (AMD) using optical coherence tomography angiography (OCTA). ***Methods:*** Literature review and case series. ***Results:*** A review of mixed neovascularization in AMD is discussed, focusing on the different subtypes of neovascularization and the associated characteristics on imaging, including fluorescein angiography, optical coherence tomography, and OCTA. Three cases are presented. ***Conclusion:*** OCTA is a method of identifying mixed neovascularization in AMD. Neovascular vessels can be seen on *en face* images of the retina, both below and above the retinal pigment epithelium, corresponding to different types of leakage observed on conventional angiography.

© 2016 S. Karger AG, Basel

Introduction

Age-related macular degeneration (AMD) is the most common cause of irreversible central vision loss in individuals over 50 years of age in the developed world [1]. Choroidal neovascularization (CNV), the hallmark of neovascular AMD, only occurs in 10–15% of these patients but is responsible for more than 80% of cases of severe visual loss [2, 3]. In these cases, abnormal blood vessels grow from the choriocapillaris and penetrate through Bruch's membrane into the subretinal pigment epithelium (RPE) (type 1 CNV) or subretinal (type 2 CNV) space [4], or they originate in the retinal layers and anastomose with the choroidal vasculature (type 3 CNV) [5]. The subsequent retinal exudation and hemorrhage cause damage to retinal tissue and can lead to disciform scarring and vision loss [6].

Fluorescein angiography (FA) and optical coherence tomography (OCT) have been and continue to be the most important imaging tests in the diagnosis and management of neovascular AMD. Optical coherence tomography angiography (OCTA) is newer to the ophthalmology armamentarium and may soon start to play a role in the management of this disease. The purpose of this chapter is to review the uses of FA and OCT in the management of neovascular AMD, focusing on mixed neovascularization, and to analyze the appearances of the different types of neovascularization in this disease on OCTA.

Imaging

Fluorescein Angiography

A variety of imaging techniques have been used to help determine disease activity in AMD. FA is useful for the identification and localization of abnormal retinal and choroidal vessels and is the current gold standard for the diagnosis of CNV in AMD [7, 8]. In addition, it can help to characterize the morphology, extent, and depth of neovascular vessels when visualized. Indocyanine green angiography (ICGA) may sometimes be combined with FA to evaluate small vessels in the deep retina and choroid to provide information on vascular permeability and ischemia [9–11].

A well-known system for CNV classification was developed for the Macular Photocoagulation Study in 1991 [12, 13]. FA was used to determine whether a CNV was classic (well defined), occult (poorly defined), or mixed in nature. With regard to each subtype, mixed lesions, usually defined as predominantly classic or minimally classic, are typically larger than occult, or type 1, lesions and have been reported to account for 10–31% of all CNV subtypes [14, 15]. In comparison, occult lesions are the most common, occurring in 60–73% of cases [15, 16]. Prior to the advent of anti-vascular endothelial growth factor (VEGF) medications, the choice of treatment with laser therapy or photodynamic therapy depended on the location, composition, and size of the lesion [12, 13, 17–19]. With the more recent use of anti-VEGF monotherapy, which is used to treat all types of neovascular AMD, the subtyping of CNV is no longer necessary.

Although FA is still commonly used to help with the diagnosis of neovascular AMD, it may be less necessary clinically due to the advent of newer noninvasive imaging techniques. Bypassing FA avoids the associated side effects of intravenous fluorescein, ranging from nausea (common) to anaphylaxis (very rare) [20, 21]. In addition, while FA can provide useful information about vascular incompetence, it penetrates poorly through hemorrhage, pigment, fibrin, and lipid [22] and provides only *en face* images, which superimpose all of the perfused layers of the retina and choroid [23].

Optical Coherence Tomography

Since its inception in the 1990s, OCT has become an essential imaging technique, and subsequent advances have allowed for the visualization of small anatomic changes within and below the retina that are associated with CNV activity [24–27]. Furthermore, as anti-VEGF medications have drastically improved the prognosis of neovascular AMD, OCT has been crucial in monitoring the response to treatment [28–32].

FA and OCT, however, provide different information regarding disease activity, and findings obtained using one imaging technique do not always correlate with those acquired using the other. Although OCT is not as well equipped to visualize retinal and choroidal blood vessels compared to FA, secondary markers of disease activity observed on OCT can be used to direct treatment without the requirement of FA. The activity of CNV on OCT is determined indirectly by the presence of subretinal fluid (SRF), intraretinal fluid, and/or retinal pigment epithelial detachment (RPED), and subretinal hyperreflective material can sometimes be seen on OCT corresponding to the CNV itself. These findings can help in the diagnosis and management of neovascular AMD without FA, avoiding the need for an invasive imaging test [33–35].

In a recent study comparing FA to the combination of FA and OCT to classify subtypes of CNV, a lower number of purely occult (type 1) lesions were diagnosed and a higher number of type 3 and 'mixed' CNV lesions were diagnosed using a combination of these two imaging techniques compared with the use of FA alone. Mixed neovascular lesions were also noted to have greater lesion areas and diameters compared to type 1 CNV lesions, which in turn had greater areas and diameters than type 2 and 3 CNV lesions [36].

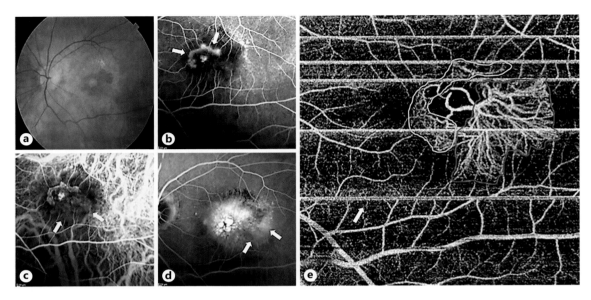

Fig. 1. a Color fundus photography demonstrates central thickening, retinal pigment epithelium (RPE) changes, and associated hemorrhage. Fluorescein angiography (FA) shows early hyperfluorescence nasally (**b**) corresponding to the classic component (arrows), and early indocyanine green angiography reveals a retinal pigment epithelial detachment (RPED) temporally (**c**) corresponding to the occult component (arrows). **d** Late FA demonstrates pooling and leakage with stippled hyperfluorescence temporally (arrows). **e** Swept-source optical coherence tomography angiography (OCTA) clearly outlines both the classic (yellow) and occult (red) components of the choroidal neovascularization (CNV). Horizontal lines corresponding to motion artifacts are seen (arrow). Images were reprinted with permission from SLACK Incorporated [43].

Optical Coherence Tomography Angiography

OCTA provides both functional information on blood flow without the need for dye injection and structural details on standard OCT B-scan images [23]. It outlines the retinal and choroidal vascular layers by detecting contrast between circulating blood cells and static tissue [37–39], and segmentation algorithms allow for the images to be separated into individual vascular beds, as presented in *en face* OCT angiograms. The outer retina is usually devoid of blood flow in healthy eyes; thus, flow detected in this area is consistent with the presence of CNV. A corresponding volumetric set of structural OCT B-scans is co-registered with *en face* OCTA images so that clinicians can visualize structure and blood flow using a single data set [39].

As OCT technology has become more advanced and images are of higher resolution and quality, CNV can often be classified based on the location of the new vessel complex on OCT [40]. Occult, or sub-epithelial (type 1), CNV is the most common subtype of neovascular AMD, while classic, or pre-epithelial (type 2), CNV is observed less frequently. Retinal angiomatous proliferation (type 3) is the least common, but structural OCT is often helpful for making the diagnosis, as the appearance of highly reflective retinal feeder vessels may be seen in association with prominent intraretinal fluid and RPED [5].

The recent introduction of OCTA to clinical practice has allowed clinicians to begin studying the different subtypes of CNV in AMD with non-invasive imaging [41–45]. Specifically, mixed-type CNV incorporates multiple types of CNV into one complex, most commonly with type 1

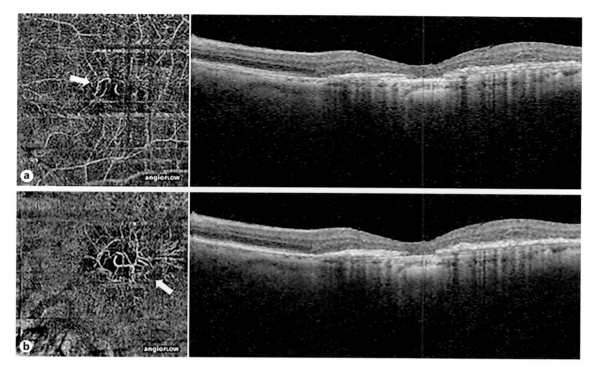

Fig. 2. a OCTA at the level of just above the RPE shows a small lacy vascular network (arrow) corresponding to the classic component. **b** Segmentation below the RPE and above Bruch's membrane allows for better visualization of the larger occult component (arrow).

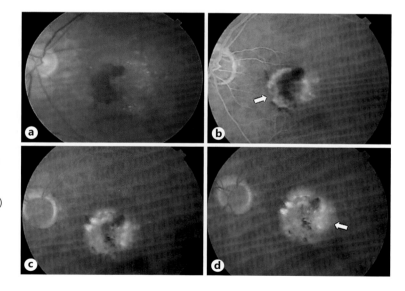

Fig. 3. a Color fundus photography shows drusen, central thickening, and hemorrhage. Early FA shows hyperfluorescence nasally (arrow, **b**) that progressively intensifies with blurring of the lesion margins (**c**). There is late pooling and leakage with temporal stippled hyperfluorescence (arrow, **d**).

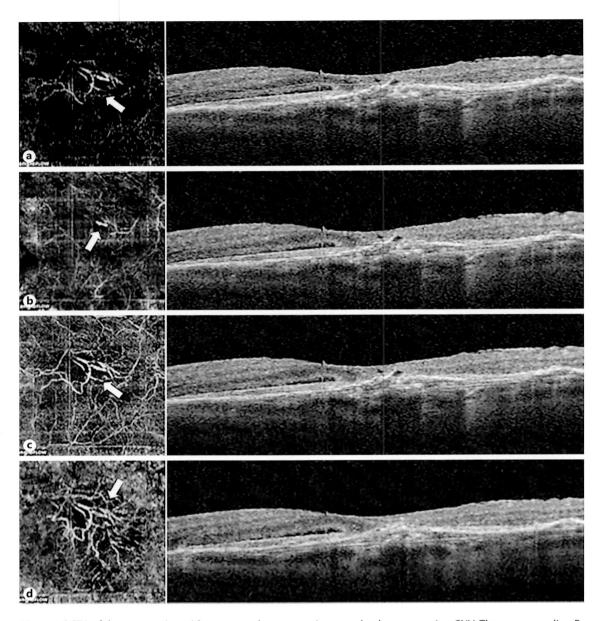

Fig. 4. a OCTA of the outer retina with automated segmentation reveals a lacy-appearing CNV. The corresponding B-scan demonstrates subretinal fluid (SRF) and subretinal hyperreflective material overlying a fibrovascular retinal RPED. Segmentation above the RPE (**b**) demonstrates a small network of vessels corresponding to the classic component of the lesion, while segmentation just below the RPE (**c**) and above Bruch's membrane (**d**) reveals the deeper and larger occult component (arrows).

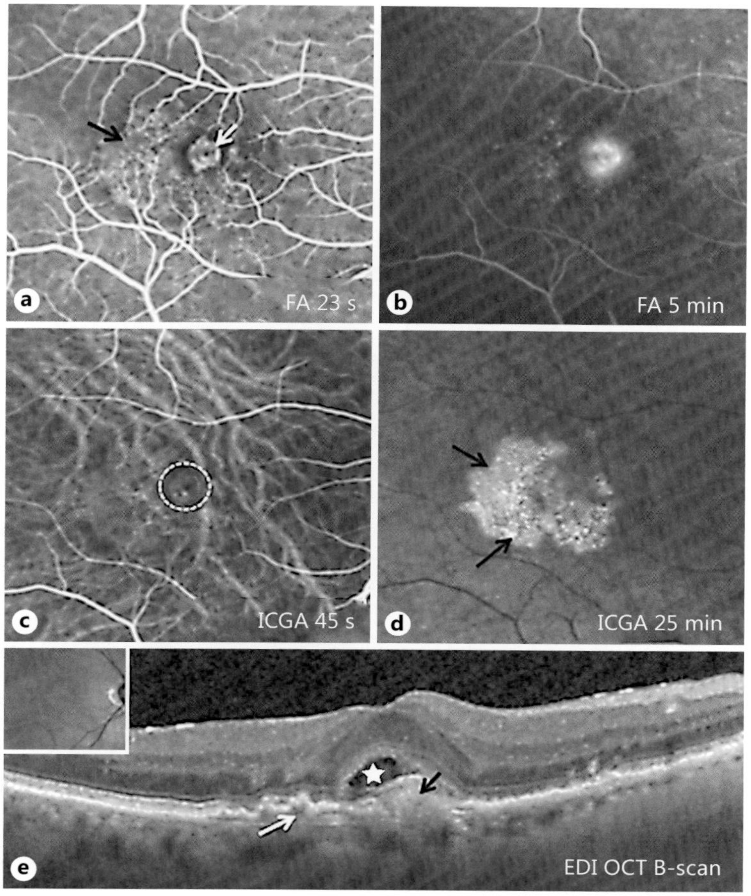

Fig. 5. a Early FA demonstrates a central hyperfluorescent lesion (white arrow) with well-defined borders and a thin hypofluorescent halo. There is an irregular hyperfluorescent area temporally (black arrow) that is representative of a fibrovascular RPED. **b** Late FA shows marked hyperfluorescence centrally with leakage and stippled hyperfluorescence temporally. Early indocyanine green angiography demonstrates a small area of rapid hyperfluorescence centrally (**c**) and late visualization of a wide neovascular network (**d**). **e** Spectral-domain optical coherence tomography imaging reveals a fibrovascular RPED with overlying SRF (white star). Image was reprinted with permission from Karger Publishers [44].

and type 2 components, and it can be visualized on both *en face* angiograms and associated B-scans.

Cases

Case 1

An 87-year-old woman presented with decreased vision in the left eye. Fundus examination revealed central thickening associated with retinal hemorrhage (fig. 1a). Early FA showed a sharply demarcated area of hyperfluorescence corresponding to the classic component of the lesion (fig. 1b), and early ICGA showed a retinal pigment epithelial detachment (RPED) corresponding to the occult component (fig. 1c). There was pooling of fluorescein on late FA that obscured the boundaries of the classic component with stippled hyperfluorescence of the occult component (fig. 1d). Swept-source OCTA clearly demonstrated both the classic (yellow) and occult (red) components of the entire CNV lesion (fig. 1e). Further segmentation of the retina above the RPE (fig. 2a) and between the RPE and Bruch's membrane (fig. 2b) on OCTA helped to visualize the classic and occult components, respectively (arrows).

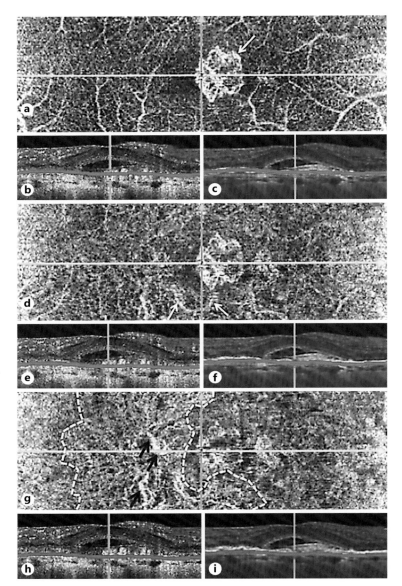

Fig. 6. OCTA at 30 microns above the RPE (**a–c**). A well-circumscribed, lacy-wheel-shaped lesion is visible on *en face* imaging representing the classic component (**a**). Corresponding B-scan images in the angio (**b**) and conventional (**c**) modes show SRF over a fibrovascular RPED. OCTA of the back surface of the RPE (**d–f**) shows that the classic lesion is still visible but is less contrasted, while another U-shaped lesion (arrows) appears. OCTA of an area deeper inside of the CNV but still above Bruch's membrane (**g–i**) reveals a larger, occult, sea fan-shaped network (dashed line). Image was reprinted with permission from Karger Publishers [44].

Case 2

An 83-year-old woman presented with decreased vision in the left eye. Fundus examination revealed drusen with central thickening and nasal hemorrhage (fig. 3a). FA showed early leakage nasally (fig. 3b) and progressive leakage in later frames (fig. 3c) with stippled hyperfluorescence temporally and pooling at the superior edge of the lesion (fig. 3d). Automated segmentation of the outer retina on OCTA demonstrated a lacy-appearing lesion, while the corresponding B-scan showed SRF overlying an area of subretinal hyperreflective material above the RPE and fibrovascular RPED (fig. 4a). Further segmentation demonstrated a small area of vessels on OCTA above the RPE corresponding to a classic component (fig. 4b), with a more visible and larger network of vessels below the RPE (fig. 4c) and closer to Bruch's membrane (fig. 4d) corresponding to the occult component.

Case 3

A 78-year-old woman presented with decreased vision in the right eye. FA (fig. 5a, b) and ICGA (fig. 5c, d) revealed a well-demarcated hyperfluorescent foveal lesion with irregular borders and a wide fibrovascular RPED component temporally. On OCT B-scan, there was retinal thickening, with SRF overlying a flat, irregular RPED (fig. 5e). OCTA of the outer retina demonstrated a well-circumscribed, lacy-wheel-shaped lesion representing classic CNV (fig. 6a–c). Further evaluation of the sub-RPE space above Bruch's membrane revealed another lesion, a U-shaped vessel that was likely draining or feeding (fig. 6d–f) and arriving from a larger network of vessels located just above Bruch's membrane (fig. 6g–i).

Conclusion

These cases demonstrate the appearance of occult (type 1) and classic (type 2) components of CNV on OCTA in neovascular AMD. While mixed types including type 3 neovascularization can also occur, they are much less common. In all three cases, the subtypes of CNV could be classified using FA and/or ICGA, but OCTA allowed for better visualization of the exact anatomy and distribution of the vascular networks both above and below the RPE, consistent with type 2 and type 1 lesions, respectively. In the management of neovascular AMD, OCTA allows for the visualization and localization of vascular networks without the need for an intravenous contrast agent, while also providing the structural details of a standard OCT B-scan.

References

1 Friedman DS, O'Colmain BJ, Muñoz B, et al: Prevalence of age-related macular degeneration in the United States. Arch Ophthalmol 2004;122:564–572.
2 Ferris FL 3rd, Fine SL, Hyman L: Age-related macular degeneration and blindness due to neovascular maculopathy. Arch Ophthalmol 1984;102:1640–1642.
3 Bressler NM: Age-related macular degeneration is the leading cause of blindness. JAMA 2004;291:1900–1901.
4 Gass J: Stereoscopic Atlas of Macular Diseases: Diagnosis and Management. St. Louis, Mosby, 1997.
5 Freund KB, Ho IV, Barbazetto IA, et al: Type 3 neovascularization: the expanded spectrum of retinal angiomatous proliferation. Retina 2008;28:201–211.
6 Ambati J, Ambati BK, Yoo SH, et al: Age-related macular degeneration: etiology, pathogenesis, and therapeutic strategies. Surv Ophthalmol 2003;48:257–293.
7 Do DV, Gower EW, Cassard SD, et al: Detection of new-onset choroidal neovascularization using optical coherence tomography: the AMD DOC Study. Ophthalmology 2012;119:771–778.

8 Do DV: Detection of new-onset choroidal neovascularization. Curr Opinion Ophthalmol 2013;24:224–227.
9 Ryan SJ, Sadda SR, Hinton DR, et al: Age-related macular degeneration; in: Ryan SJ (ed): Retina. China, Saunders, 2013, pp 1150–1582.
10 Shah SM, Tatlipinar S, Quinlan E, et al: Dynamic and quantitative analysis of choroidal neovascularization by fluorescein angiography. Invest Ophthalmol Vis Sci 2006;47:5460–5468.
11 Sulzbacher F, Kiss C, Munk M, et al: Diagnostic evaluation of type 2 (classic) choroidal neovascularization: optical coherence tomography, indocyanine green angiography, and fluorescein angiography. Am J Ophthalmol 2011;152: 799–806.
12 Macular Photocoagulation Study Group: Laser photocoagulation of subfoveal neovascular lesions in age-related macular degeneration. Results of a randomized clinical trial. Arch Ophthalmol 1991;109:1220–1231.

13 Macular Photocoagulation Study Group: Occult choroidal neovascularization. Influence on visual outcome in patients with age-related macular degeneration. Arch Ophthalmol 1996;114:400–412.
14 Beaumont PE, Kang HK: Lesion morphology in age-related macular degeneration and its therapeutic significance. Arch Ophthalmol 2006;124:807–812.
15 Bermig J, Tylla H, Jochmann C, et al: Angiographic findings in patients with exudative age-related macular degeneration. Graefes Arch Clin Exp Ophthalmol 2002;240:169–175.
16 Olsen TW, Feng X, Kasper TJ, et al: Fluorescein angiographic lesion type frequency in neovascular age-related macular degeneration. Ophthalmology 2004; 111:250–255.
17 Treatment of Age-Related Macular Degeneration with Photodynamic Therapy (TAP) Study Group: Photodynamic therapy of subfoveal choroidal neovascularization in age-related macular degeneration with verteporfin: two-year results of 2 randomized clinical trials–TAP report 2. Arch Ophthalmol 2001;119:198–207.

18 Verteporfin in Photodynamic Therapy Study Group: Verteporfin therapy of subfoveal choroidal neovascularization in age-related macular degeneration: two-year results of a randomized clinical trial including lesions with occult with no classic choroidal neovascularization–verteporfin in photodynamic therapy report 2. Am J Ophthalmol 2001;131: 541–560.

19 Barbazetto I, Burdan A, Bressler NM, et al: Photodynamic therapy of subfoveal choroidal neovascularization with verteporfin: fluorescein angiographic guidelines for evaluation and treatment–TAP and VIP report No. 2. Arch Ophthalmol 2003;121:1253–1268.

20 Kwiterovich KA, Maguire MG, Murphy RP, et al: Frequency of adverse systemic reactions after fluorescein angiography. Results of a prospective study. Ophthalmology 1991;98:1139–1142.

21 Lopez-Saez MP, Ordoqui E, Tornero P, et al: Fluorescein-induced allergic reaction. Ann Allergy Asthma Immunol 1998;81:428–430.

22 Jia Y, Bailey ST, Hwang TS, et al: Quantitative optical coherence tomography angiography of vascular abnormalities in the living human eye. Proc Natl Acad Sci U S A 2015;112:E2395–E2402.

23 Coscas G, Lupidi M, Coscas F: Atlas of OCT-Angiography in AMD: Comparison with Multimodal Imaging. Paris, Créteil, Perugia, 2015.

24 Rosenfeld PJ, Moshfeghi AA, Puliafito CA: Optical coherence tomography findings after an intravitreal injection of bevacizumab (Avastin) for neovascular age-related macular degeneration. Ophthalmic Surg Lasers 2005;36: 331–335.

25 Kaiser PK, Blodi BA, Shapiro H, et al: Angiographic and optical coherence tomographic results of the MARINA study of ranibizumab in neovascular age-related macular degeneration. Ophthalmology 2007;114:1868–1875.

26 Fung AE, Lalwani GA, Rosenfeld PJ, et al: An optical coherence tomography-guided, variable dosing regimen with intravitreal ranibizumab (Lucentis) for neovascular age related macular degeneration. Am J Ophthalmol 2007;143: 566–583.

27 Lalwani GA, Rosenfeld PJ, Fung AE, et al: A variable-dosing regimen with intravitreal ranibizumab for neovascular age-related macular degeneration: year 2 of the PrONTO Study. Am J Ophthalmol 2009;148:43–58.

28 Avery RL, Pieramici DJ, Rabena MD, et al: Intravitreal bevacizumab (Avastin) for neovascular age-related macular degeneration. Ophthalmology 2006;113: 363–372.

29 Rosenfeld PJ, Brown DM, Heier JS, et al: Ranibizumab for neovascular age-related macular degeneration. N Engl J Med 2006;355:1419–1431.

30 Schmidt-Erfurth UM, Pruente C: Management of neovascular age-related macular degeneration. Prog Retin Eye Res 2007;26:437–451.

31 CATT Research Group, Martin DF, Maguire MG, et al: Ranibizumab and bevacizumab for neovascular age-related macular degeneration. N Engl J Med 2011;364:1897–1908.

32 Heier JS, Brown DM, Chong V, et al: Intravitreal aflibercept (VEGF trap-eye) in wet age-related macular degeneration. Ophthalmology 2012;119:2537–2548.

33 Liakopolous S, Ongchin S, Bansal A, et al: Quantitative optical coherence tomography findings in various subtypes of neovascular age-related macular degeneration. Invest Ophthalmol Vis Sci 2008;49:5048–5054.

34 Sadda SR, Liakopolous S, Keane PA, et al: Relationship between angiographic and optical coherence tomographic (OCT) parameters for quantifying choroidal neovascular lesions. Graefes Arch Clin Exp Ophthalmol 2010;248:175–184.

35 Giant A, Luiselli C, Esmaili DD, et al: Spectral-domain optical coherence tomography as an indicator of fluorescein angiography leakage from choroidal neovascularization. Retina 2011;52: 5579–5586.

36 Jung JJ, Chen CY, Mrejen S, et al: The incidence of neovascular subtypes in newly diagnosed neovascular age-related macular degeneration. Am J Ophthalmol 2014;158:769–779.

37 Zawinka C, Ergun E, Stur M: Prevalence of patients presenting with neovascular age-related macular degeneration in an urban population. Retina 2005;25:324–331.

38 Spaide RF, Klancnik JM Jr, Cooney MJ: Retinal vascular layers imaged by fluorescein angiography and optical coherence tomography angiography. JAMA Ophthalmol 2015;133:45–50.

39 Jia Y, Bailey ST, Wilson DJ, et al: Quantitative optical coherence tomography angiography of choroidal neovascularization in age-related macular degeneration. Ophthalmol 2014;121:1435–1444.

40 Freund KB, Zweifel SA, Engelbert M: Do we need a new classification for choroidal neovascularization in age-related macular degeneration? Retina 2010;30: 1333–1349.

41 Kuehlewein L, Bansal M, Lenis T, et al: Optical coherence tomography angiography of type 1 neovascularization in age-related macular degeneration. Am J Ophthalmol 2015;160:739–748.

42 Kuehlewein L, Sadda SR, Sarraf D: OCT angiography and sequential quantitative analysis of type 2 neovascularization after ranibizumab therapy. Eye (Lond) 2015;29:932–935.

43 Moult E, Choi W, Waheed NK, et al: Ultrahigh-speed swept-source OCT angiography in exudative AMD. Ophthalmic Surg Lasers Imaging Retina 2014; 45:496–505.

44 Coscas G, Lupidi M, Coscas F, et al: Optical coherence tomography angiography during follow up: qualitative and quantitative analysis of mixed type I and II choroidal neovascularization after vascular endothelial growth factor trap therapy. Ophthalmic Res 2015;54:57–63.

45 Dansingani KK, Naysan J, Freund KB: En face OCT angiography demonstrates flow in early type 3 neovascularization (retinal angiomatous proliferation). Eye (Lond) 2015;29:703–706.

Andre J. Witkin, MD
New England Eye Center
800 Washington Street, Box 450
Boston, MA 02111 (USA)
E-Mail awitkin@tuftsmedicalcenter.org

Bandello F, Souied EH, Querques G (eds): OCT Angiography in Retinal and Macular Diseases.
Dev Ophthalmol. Basel, Karger, 2016, vol 56, pp 71–76 (DOI: 10.1159/000442781)

Optical Coherence Tomography Angiography of Idiopathic Polypoidal Choroidal Vasculopathy

Mayer Srour[a] · Giuseppe Querques[a, b] · Eric H. Souied[a]

[a]Department of Ophthalmology, Centre Hospitalier Intercommunal de Créteil, Universite Paris Est Créteil, Créteil, France;
[b]Department of Ophthalmology IRCCS San Raffaele Scientific Institute University Vita-Salute San Raffaele, Milan, Italy

Abstract

Purpose: To analyze the morphological characteristics of polypoidal choroidal vasculopathy (PCV) on optical coherence tomography angiography (OCT-A). ***Methods:*** Consecutive patients with PCV underwent complete ophthalmological examination, including fundus photography, fluorescein angiography, indocyanine green angiography, spectral-domain OCT and OCT-A. ***Results:*** Segmentation of the choriocapillaris layer on OCT-A revealed the branching vascular network as a hyper-flow lesion, and it revealed the polypoidal lesion as a hyper-flow round structure surrounded by a hypo-intense halo in some cases and as a hypo-flow round structure in most cases. ***Conclusion:*** OCT-A is a noninvasive imaging modality that allows for the visualization of different structures in PCV. The branching vascular network is consistently and clearly detected. The hypo-flow round appearance of the polyps on OCT-A is probably due to unusual blood flow inside of the polypoidal lesions, in contrast with the branching vascular network. Further improvements in OCT-A knowledge will provide information on the specificity of the different intensity characteristics in PCV.

© 2016 S. Karger AG, Basel

Polypoidal choroidal vasculopathy (PCV) is an acquired, abnormal choroidal vasculopathy that is distinct from typical choroidal neovascularization [1, 2]. PCV was first described in 1982 by Yannuzzi (Yannuzzi LA. Idiopathic polypoidal choroidal vasculopathy. Macula Society Meeting 1982; Miami, Fla., USA).

PCV is characterized by polypoidal dilations and choroidal branching vascular networks observed on indocyanine green angiography (ICGA) [1–4]. Optical coherence tomography (OCT) is a very useful tool for the diagnosis of PCV, as polypoidal dilations are characterized by dome-like

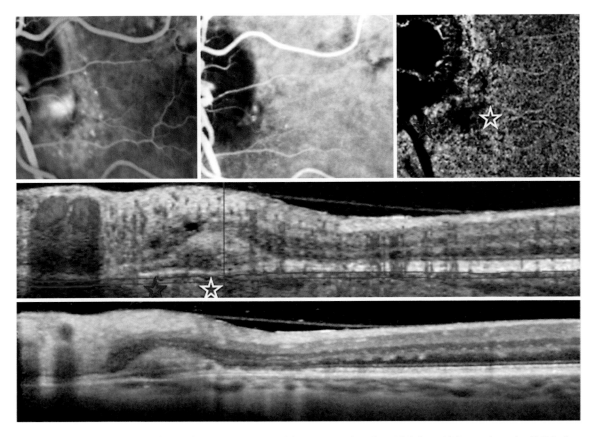

Fig. 1. Multimodal imaging of the left eye of a 65-year-old woman with polypoidal choroidal vasculopathy (PCV) after 9 intravitreal anti-VEGF injections and 1 half-fluence photodynamic therapy session 6 months prior. Fluorescein angiography (top left), indocyanine green angiography (ICGA) (top middle) and spectral-domain optical coherence tomography (OCT) (bottom) images, showing the polypoidal lesion and corresponding abnormal choroidal vascular network. Optical coherence tomography angiography (OCT-A) image of the choriocapillaris segmentation (double red line) with the corresponding OCT B-scan (top right, middle), revealing the branching vascular network as a hyperflow lesion (blue star) and the polypoidal lesion as hypo-flow round structure (white star). A comparison of the OCT-A and ICGA images reveals that the OCT-A characteristics of PCV correspond topographically to the branching vascular network and polypoidal lesions visualized on ICGA.

elevations of retinal pigment epithelium and moderate internal reflectivity [5–7]. Branching vascular networks appear on OCT images as two highly reflective lines ('double layer sign') [8].

Optical coherence tomography angiography (OCT-A) is an emerging imaging technique that allows for blood flow visualization by means of the split-spectrum amplitude-decorrelation angiography algorithm (among other technologies) [9, 10].

Consecutive patients with PCV underwent complete ophthalmological examination, including fundus photography, fluorescein angiography, ICGA, spectral-domain OCT and OCT-A.

An OCT-A image of the choriocapillaris segmentation revealed the branching vascular network as a hyper-flow lesion (fig. 1–4) and the polypoidal lesion as a hypo-flow round structure in most cases (fig. 1, 4), but in some cases, the

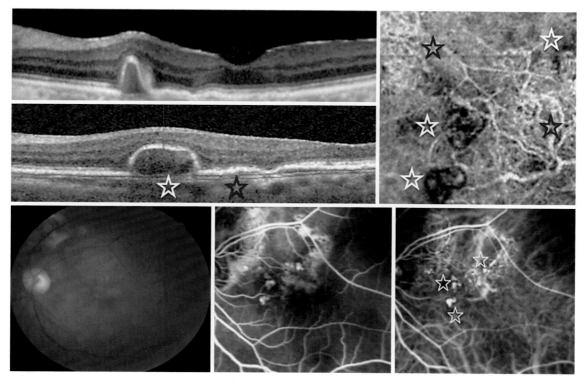

Fig. 2. Multimodal imaging of the left eye of a 67-year-old Asian woman with PCV after 13 intravitreal anti-VEGF injections. Fundus (bottom left), fluorescein angiography (bottom middle), ICGA (bottom right), and spectral-domain OCT (top left) images, showing the polypoidal lesion and corresponding abnormal choroidal vascular network. Note that on ICGA, three hyperfluorescent round structures (white stars) are present corresponding to polypoidal lesions. OCT-A image of the choriocapillaris segmentation (double red line) and the corresponding B-scan (middle left, top right) reveal the branching vascular network as a hyper-flow lesion (blue star) and the three polypoidal lesions as hyper-flow round structures surrounded by a hypo-intense halo (white star). A comparison of the OCT-A and ICGA images reveals that the OCT-A characteristics of PCV correspond topographically to the branching vascular network and polypoidal lesions visualized on ICGA.

polypoidal lesion appeared as a hyper-flow round structure surrounded by a hypo-intense halo (fig. 2, 3). A comparison of OCT-A and ICGA images revealed that the OCT-A characteristics of PCV corresponded topographically to the branching vascular network and polypoidal lesions visualized on ICGA (fig. 1–4).

Polypoidal lesions characteristically appear as hypo-flow round structures on OCT-A. However, this absence of signal does not mean that there is no blood flow; rather, it indicates that blood flow is not within the detection limit of the

OCT-A device. This could be due to either increased or decreased flow in the polyps and subsequent nonvisualization of the vascular structure. Although choroidal blood flow is known to be higher than retinal blood flow [11], and some studies of PCV hemodynamics have suggested that these lesions originate from choroidal vascularization [12], this hypothesis is very unlikely. High blood flow in the polyps is theoretically possible, but ICGA has revealed that the polyps do not fill very rapidly during early-phase angiography.

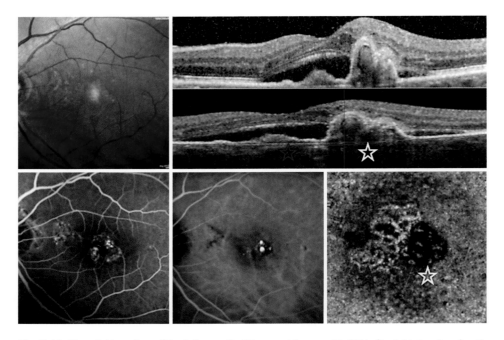

Fig. 3. Multimodal imaging of the left eye of a 66-year-old man with PCV after 12 intravitreal anti-VEGF injections and 1 half-fluence photodynamic therapy session 3 months prior. Multicolor imaging (top left), fluorescein angiography (bottom left), ICGA (bottom middle) and spectral-domain OCT (top right) images, showing the polypoidal lesion and corresponding abnormal choroidal vascular network. OCT-A image of the choriocapillaris segmentation (double red line) and the corresponding B-scan (top right, middle right) reveal the branching vascular network as a hyper-flow lesion (blue star) and the polypoidal lesion as a hyper-flow round structure surrounded by a hypo-intense halo (white star). A comparison of the OCT-A and ICGA images reveals that the OCT-A characteristics of PCV correspond topographically to the branching vascular network and polypoidal lesions visualized on ICGA.

We hypothesize that the apparent absence of OCT-A signal within polypoidal lesions could be due to either the presence of turbulent blood flow inside of the polyps – impeding the representation of this flow – or to the fact that blood circulates only at the periphery of the aneurysmal dilation. The last hypothesis is sustained by the fact that the pigmentary epithelium detachment associated with the polypoidal structure also demonstrates an attenuated OCT-A signal.

As some of our patients with PCV who were imaged using OCT-A were previously treated, we hypothesize that the various structural OCT-A aspects of polyps can be explained by the effect of anti-VEGF treatment or photodynamic therapy on blood flow. Miura et al. [13] have demonstrated that composite Doppler OCT B-scan images show the presence of blood flow inside of polypoidal lesions and the disappearance or reduction of blood flow after treatment, probably due to changes in polyp structure with obstruction of the vessel wall by a thrombus or by a phenomenon of hyalinization [14]. Moreover, we cannot exclude that the appearance of the polyps as hyper-flow round structures surrounded by a hypo-intense halo, as sometimes observed on OCT-A, could be related to artifact phenomena caused by the projection of retinal vessels [15].

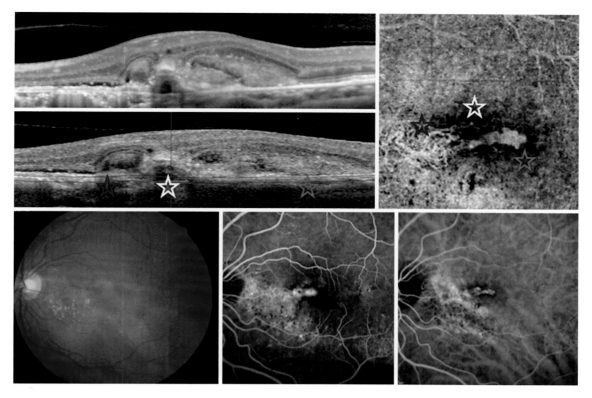

Fig. 4. Multimodal imaging of the left eye of a 67-year-old woman with PCV associated with classic (type 2) choroidal neovascularization (CNV) naïve to treatment. Fundus (bottom left), fluorescein angiography (bottom middle), ICGA (bottom right) and spectral-domain OCT (top left) images, showing the polypoidal lesion and corresponding abnormal choroidal vascular network associated with classic CNV. OCT-A image of the choriocapillaris segmentation (double red line) and the corresponding OCT B-scan (middle left, top right) reveal the branching vascular network as a hyper-flow lesion (blue star) and the polypoidal lesion as a hypo-flow round structure (white star). The classic CNV appears as a hyper-flow structure (red star). A comparison of the OCT-A and ICGA images reveals that the OCT-A characteristics of PCV correspond topographically to the branching vascular network and polypoidal lesions visualized on ICGA.

OCT-A allows for the visualization of retinal microvasculature by detecting intravascular linear blood flow [9, 10], and indeed, in our patients, the branching vascular network, which is characterized by linear blood flow, was clearly detected using the split-spectrum amplitude-decorrelation angiography algorithm.

OCT-A is a noninvasive imaging modality, and we have demonstrated that it allows for the visualization of different structures in PCV. The branching vascular networks are clearly and consistently visualized as hyper-flow lesions, but further improvements in OCT-A knowledge are needed to gather information on the specificity of the different intensity characteristics of polypoidal lesions.

References

1 Yannuzzi LA, Sorenson J, Spaide RF, et al: Idiopathic polypoidal choroidal vasculopathy (IPCV). Retina (Philadelphia, Pa.) 1990;10:1–8.

2 Laude A, Cackett PD, Vithana EN, et al: Polypoidal choroidal vasculopathy and neovascular age-related macular degeneration: same or different disease? Prog Retin Eye Res 2010;29:19–29.

3 Ciardella AP, Donsoff IM, Huang SJ, et al: Polypoidal choroidal vasculopathy. Surv Ophthalmol 2004;49:25–37.

4 Spaide RF, Yannuzzi LA, Slakter JS, et al: Indocyanine green videoangiography of idiopathic polypoidal choroidal vasculopathy. Retina (Philadelphia, Pa.) 1995; 15:100–110.

5 Sa H-S, Cho HY, Kang SW: Optical coherence tomography of idiopathic polypoidal choroidal vasculopathy. Korean J Ophthalmol 2005;19:275–280.

6 Iijima H, Imai M, Gohdo T, et al: Optical coherence tomography of idiopathic polypoidal choroidal vasculopathy. Am J Ophthalmol 1999;127:301–305.

7 Otsuji T, Takahashi K, Fukushima I, et al: Optical coherence tomographic findings of idiopathic polypoidal choroidal vasculopathy. Ophthalmic Surg Lasers 2000;31:210–214.

8 Sato T, Kishi S, Watanabe G, et al: Tomographic features of branching vascular networks in polypoidal choroidal vasculopathy. Retina (Philadelphia, Pa.) 2007;27:589–594.

9 Jia Y, Tan O, Tokayer J, et al: Split-spectrum amplitude-decorrelation angiography with optical coherence tomography. Opt Express 2012;20:4710–4725.

10 Jia Y, Bailey ST, Wilson DJ, et al: Quantitative optical coherence tomography angiography of choroidal neovascularization in age-related macular degeneration. Ophthalmology 2014;121:1435–1444.

11 Muir ER, Duong TQ: MRI of retinal and choroidal blood flow with laminar resolution. NMR Biomed 2011;24:216–223.

12 Watanabe G, Fujii H, Kishi S: Imaging of choroidal hemodynamics in eyes with polypoidal choroidal vasculopathy using laser speckle phenomenon. Jpn J Ophthalmol 2008;52:175–181.

13 Miura M, Muramatsu D, Hong Y-J, et al: Noninvasive vascular imaging of polypoidal choroidal vasculopathy by Doppler optical coherence tomography. Invest Ophthalmol Vis Sci 2015;56:3179–3186.

14 Nakashizuka H, Mitsumata M, Okisaka S, et al: Clinicopathologic findings in polypoidal choroidal vasculopathy. Invest Ophthalmol Vis Sci 2008;49:4729–4737.

15 Spaide RF, Fujimoto JG, Waheed NK: Image artifacts in optical coherence tomography angiography. Retina 2015;35:2163–2180.

Eric H. Souied
Department of Ophthalmology, Centre Hospitalier Intercommunal de Créteil
Universite Paris Est Créteil, 40 Avenue de Verdun
FR–94000 Créteil (France)
E-Mail eric.souied@chicreteil.fr

Bandello F, Souied EH, Querques G (eds): OCT Angiography in Retinal and Macular Diseases.
Dev Ophthalmol. Basel, Karger, 2016, vol 56, pp 77–85 (DOI: 10.1159/000442782)

Optical Coherence Tomography Angiography Study of Choroidal Neovascularization Early Response after Treatment

Bruno Lumbroso[a] · Marco Rispoli[a] · Maria Cristina Savastano[a] · Yali Jia[b] · Ou Tan[b] · David Huang[b]

[a]Centro Italiano Macula, Rome, Italy; [b]Casey Eye Institute, Oregon Health and Science University, Portland, Oreg., USA

Abstract

Aims: Study the choroidal neovascularization (CNV) morphological evolution after treatment using optical coherence tomography angiography (OCTA). ***Method:*** We used Optovue XR Avanti, with split-spectrum amplitude-decorrelation angiography algorithm. ***Results:*** OCT Angiography allows to recognize better the CNV type. In our series all our cases seem to follow a 45 to 60 days cycle, after intra vitreal injection. After each injection a pruning of smaller vessels is seen immediately (after 24 hours) that increases for 6 to 12 days when it reaches a maximum. It is followed by a reopening or new sprouting of the vessels 20 to 50 days later. The later cycles seem longer. Our results on early CNV evolution seem to confirm previous observations of CNV abnormalization and arterialization. Pruning the small peripheral branches seems to strengthen the trunk. In OCTA, closing terminal vessels (anti-VEGF effects) seems to cause an increased flow in trunk after the CNV reactivation.   © 2016 S. Karger AG, Basel

Over the last 2 years, our groups from Rome and Portland have been interested in the morphological changes during the early evolution of choroidal neovascularization (CNV) vessels that develop days and weeks after treatment with repeated intravitreous anti-vascular endothelial growth factor (VEGF) injections, as visualized on optical coherence tomography angiography (OCTA). Fluorescein angiography (FA) and indocyanine green angiography [1, 2] have been used until very recently for the study of CNV, but they do not allow for precise visualization of new vascular vessels, only of their indistinct margins, due to early dye leakage. The use of OCTA to examine CNV provides images that are similar to early indocyanine green angiography images, but vessel features appear sharper. It is possible to easily recognize the feeder vessel or vessels and the collateral branches, with anastomoses and loops. CNV is a complex process that occurs from early onset, over the evolution of the disease with or without treatment, and finally culminates in fibrosis and atrophy [3, 4].

Two years ago, a new tool for evaluating retinal circulation without the use of dye was introduced [5]. It is based on split-spectrum amplitude-decorrelation angiography, and it allows for the visualization of flow detection and connectivity of the retinal microvascular network. This new method has been termed OCTA [6]. As reported by De Carlo, Duker, and Waheed et al. [7] OCTA shows all CNV features better and more easily without causing adverse effects.

Studies using OCTA to examine CNV evolution after treatment are rare. Spaide [8] reported the long-term evolution of type I CNV in 17 eyes of patients followed for years who received a mean of 47 injections. De Carlo, Duker, and Waheed et al. [3] reported one patient followed up at 1 week, 3 weeks, and 2 months after injection with anti-VEGF. Kuehlewein et al. [9] described one patient who received OCTA 4 weeks after the first ranibizumab injection and 2 and 4 weeks after the second injection.

Angiogenesis is crucial to the physiopathology of CNV and is a progressive process that causes vessel proliferation. As first reported by Ferrara [10] and then by Spaide [8], the angiogenesis process is highly affected by anti-VEGF treatment. VEGF is considered to be the main target in the treatment of vasoproliferative diseases, and angiogenesis is VEGF-dependent. Two mechanisms operate in the development of neovascularization: *arteriogenesis*, which results in dilatation of the preexisting channel, and *angiogenesis,* which promotes the sprouting of new vessels.

Our groups of Lumbroso, Rispoli, and Savastano from Rome and Huang, Jia, and Tan from Portland have observed the morphological changes that occur during the early evolution of vessels at days and weeks after treatment with repeated intravitreous anti-VEGF injections using OCTA. They performed OCTA at 24 h after injection and then 7, 20 and 30 days later. All of the patients agreed willingly to receive these frequently repeated OCTAs. We have recently published our results: Lumbroso et al. [11] and Huang et al. [12]. In this chapter, we report two new cases that were not included in our 2015 Retina articles [11, 12] and the conclusions that could be drawn. We assessed early CNV modifications that occurred af-

ter intravitreal therapy, even after a duration of as short as 24 h after treatment, by OCTA. During follow-up, it is now possible using OCTA to pinpoint CNV regions that remain unchanged or that do not go through significant changes and other regions that vary or seem to disappear for some time.

Methods and Technique

In this observational longitudinal study, a total of 7 eyes from 7 patients with naïve CNV type 2 were assessed by OCTA. This CNV series included 5 cases of classic type 2 CNV, one case of type 2 CNV in a fibrovascular formation, and one case of mixed types 1 and 2. On OCT B-scans, type 2 CNV was defined by the presence of retinal edema and no retinal pigment epithelium (RPE) elevation, and a mixture of types 1 and 2 CNV was identified by the presence of a hyperreflective subretinal formation anterior to an elevated, disrupted RPE.

OCTA was performed to closely observe the *early evolution of neovascularization* after intravitreal aflibercept or ranibizumab injection precisely at 24 h, 7–10 days, 12–18 days and 28–35 days after injection. The loading phase interval was about 30 days. The follow-up times were between 10 and 18 months.

The OCTA instrument used was based on an AngioVue Imaging System (Optovue, Inc., Freemont, Calif., USA) used for obtaining amplitude-decorrelation angiography images. This instrument has an A-scan rate of 70,000 scans per s, using a light source centered on 840 nm and a bandwidth of 50 nm. Each OCTA volume includes 304 × 304 A-scans with two consecutive B-scans captured at each fixed position before proceeding to the next sampling location. Split-spectrum amplitude-decorrelation angiography was used to extract the OCTA information. Each OCTA volume was acquired in 3 s, and two orthogonal OCTA volumes were acquired to perform motion correction to minimize motion artifacts arising from microsaccades and fixation changes. The angiography data presented was the average of the decorrelation values for perpendicular views through the region being evaluated. The macular angiography scan protocol covered a 3 × 3 mm area. The stack of angiography images selected was applied to visualize the neovascularization, and an automated change analysis protocol was applied during follow-up.

OCTA software was used to delineate the region of interest. The inner and outer boundaries of OCT angiograms included all apparent CNV vessels. An artifact removal option in the software allowed for the subtracting of retinal vessel reflection (derived from RPE reflection) from flow images. Two independent readers examined the OCTA scans, with agreement of >92%.

The research performed in this study adhered to the tenets of the Declaration of Helsinki.

Results

In this observational longitudinal study of 7 eyes from 7 patients with a mean age of 74.5 (±15.12) years, including 6 women and one man (all naïve cases) were followed from 10 to 18 months, and over that time, they had a mean of 5.5 intravitreal injections (ranging from 3 to 8) and a mean of 10 OCTA examinations each (ranging from 8 to 26).

CNV morphology was assessed in all eyes followed from 10 to 18 months (about 20 cycles), with OCTA performed at 24 h, 7–10 days, 12–18 days and 28–35 days after injection treatment, and 3–4 controls were used per month.

Recurring Choroidal Neovascularization Evolution

The morphology of CNV after injection seemed to change with time as follows:

24 h after treatment: the number of visible vessels decreased, with apparent vessel fragmentation. The CNV area decreased, with pruning of thinner anastomoses and the loss of small vessels. Residual flow was uneven and was more evident close to the afferent trunk, with important microvascular rarefaction, decreased vessel caliber, and vessel narrowing. The CNV area and vessel density decreased due to the loss of smaller vessels.

7–10 days after injection: the number of visible vessels and CNV area continued to decrease. The remaining surviving vessels were grouped around the feeder trunk.

12–18 days after injection: the maximum decrease in the number of vessels was observed.

28–35 days after injection: reproliferation was detected. The vessels had approximately the same appearance as they had before treatment and collapse, but the vessel caliber was greater, and the CNV area was smaller. The number of thinner capillaries decreased, but some anastomoses and loops reappeared.

After 5–8 cycles of 60–70 days: the vessels were thicker and straighter, with increased flow, and features of arterialization were detected (table 1).

After 5–10 cycles of 60–70 days: the vessels were fewer in number, thicker, and straighter, with increased flow, and apparent arterialization was observed.

During the loading phase, three intravitreal injections were supposed to be administered at 30-day intervals. In our clinic, it was not possible to strictly follow this protocol. The mean interval was 39 days, without counting one patient who came back after 70 days.

Periodic Evolution

The cycle mean duration during the loading phase was 42.5 days (11 cycles ranged from 34 to 70 days). After the loading phase, we followed a pro re nata (PRN; as-needed) treatment regimen. Retreatment was applied in the case of recurrence of fluid accumulation, before recurrence of metamorphopsia and before a further decrease in visual acuity.

Once again, in our clinic, it was not possible to strictly follow this protocol. During this short observational period, we did not observe retinal bleeding. In the few cases in which the injection was administered later than a few days after the observation of activity, metamorphopsia and visual acuity changes were observed.

Table 1. Features of choroidal neovascularization type 2 after anti-VEGF injection on OCTA

At 24 h	Decreased CNV area Decreased vessel density Loss of smaller vessels Reduced number of anastomoses Microvascular rarefaction Reduction of vessel diameter and vessel narrowing Apparent vessel fragmentation
At day 7–10 days	Further decrease in number of visible vessels Further decrease in CNV area, with unchanged or slightly smaller central CNV feeder
At day 12–18 days	Maximum decrease in number of visible vessels
At day 28–35 days	Vessels reproliferation begins
At 35–40 days	Vessel reproliferation. Some preexisting main vessels reappear and are thicker and straighter with increased flow

The cycle mean duration after the loading phase was 62.3 days (9 cycles ranged from 34 to 107 days). After 5–8 cycles of 60–70 days, the vessels appeared to be fewer in number, thicker, and straighter, with increased flow. These changes appeared to result in arterialization with a decreased CNV area, a decreased vessel density, loss of smaller vessels, and a reduction in the number of anastomoses.

The vessel diameters were increased and larger.

We report two cases that were not included in our 2015 Retina articles [11, 12] and the conclusions that can be drawn.

Case Evolution

Evolution of Case 1 with Type 2 Choroidal Neovascularization in Age-Related Macular Degeneration
An 81-year-old woman came to our office for metamorphopsia in the right eye lasting for several weeks. Upon examination, she was emmetropic, with vision of 70 and 90 ETDRS letters in the right and left eyes, respectively. Cross-section OCT showed cystoid macular edema. FA and OCTA showed type 2 CNV in the left eye and no drusen in the right eye. The CNV was close to the fovea, with a central afferent vessel and dense capillary arborescence. A dark area was seen around the CNV.

First Treatment, First Cycle
Twenty-Four Hours after Treatment: OCTA showed a neat decrease in the number of visible vessels, with no apparent vessel fragmentation. The CNV area was smaller. The vessels that were still visible were decreased in number and density, with the pruning of thinner anastomoses and loss of smaller vessels. The network density was decreased, with only some major preexisting vessels highlighted. Residual flow was uneven and was more visible close to the afferent trunk. The results were as follows: an important loss of smaller vessels, microvascular rarefaction, decreased vessel caliber, and vessel narrowing.
Seven Days after Injection: the number of remaining surviving vessels decreased and were grouped together around the feeder vessel.
Thirty-Two Days after Injection: no reproliferated vessels were seen. The CNV area was clearly smaller. The visible vessels on OCTA were thicker and straighter, with loss of smaller vessels. The decreases in the CNV area and vessel density were due to the loss of smaller capillaries.

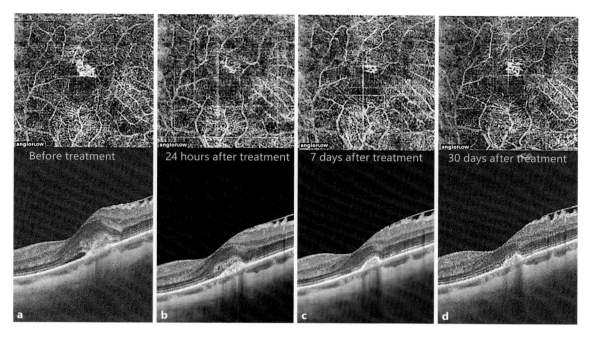

Fig. 1. First cycle after treatment of naïve choroidal neovascularization (CNV); evolution of Case 1, an 81-year-old woman with type 2 CNV in age-related macular degeneration. **a** Optical coherence tomography angiography (OCTA) shows type 2 CNV close to the fovea, with a central afferent vessel and dense capillary arborescence. A dark area is seen around the CNV. **b** Twenty-four hours after treatment: OCTA shows a neat decrease in the number of visible vessels. The CNV area is smaller, with an important loss of smaller vessels, microvascular rarefaction, decreased vessel caliber, and vessel narrowing. **c** Seven days after injection: the number of remaining vessels decrease and are grouped around the feeder vessel. **d** Thirty-two days after injection: the CNV area is smaller. The vessels are thicker and straighter with the loss of smaller vessels on OCTA.

A second treatment was performed at 45 days after the first treatment (second cycle).

2° Cycle – 24 Hours after Treatment: the number of visible vessels decreased, and pruning of thinner anastomoses was observed. Residual flow was more visible close to the feeder vessel.

2° Cycle – 18 Days after Injection: reproliferating vessels appeared with a greater vessel caliber, and the loss of smaller vessels was observed.

After Third and Fourth Injections: the CNV area was smaller but denser with increased flow. Fewer vessels reappeared, and they had *larger diameters* and were straighter; in addition, there was an increased loss of smaller vessels. The CNV mean area and vessel density were smaller, but some anastomoses reappeared.

After each new treatment, the same main vessels seemed to reappear, with increased flow and decreased branch density. The CNV area was smaller. Some main branches did not seem to be affected by the treatment. Some new vessels sprouted in new areas, and in other areas, small capillaries reopened.

This evolution is similar to that described by Spaide, and it seems to confirm his theory of CNV *abnormalization* after treatment [8]. Following further treatments, the same vessels seemed to reappear with increased flow and decreased branch density. Some small tufts of new sprouting seemed to originate from the main branches (fig. 1).

The dark choriocapillaris area around the CNV remains apparently unchanged throughout disease evolution.

Evolution of Case 2 with Type 2 Choroidal Neovascularization in Fibrotic Formation in Age-Related Macular Degeneration

An 80-year-old man came to our office for a decrease in vision and no metamorphopsia in his left eye. Upon examination, he was emmetropic, with vision in the left eye of 75 ETDRS letters.

Slit lamp examination showed a well-demarcated, slightly elevated small mass of dark yellow tissue at the fovea.

A cross-section scan showed retinal elevation and a dense square-shaped hyperreflective elongated mass adherent to the RPE. There was some subretinal fluid and possible losses of the adjacent RPE and ellipsoid zone. These features are indicative of type 2 CNV.

OCTA showed CNV in the left eye inside of a horizontal ovoid formation, with a dark choriocapillaris ring-shaped area around the fibrotic formation. The deep, dark area was probably related to the masking effect generated by the fibrous tissue.

An irregular, fragmented neovascular network was seen inside of the fibrotic tissue. The vessels appeared as a tangled network with small branches, a few vascular loops and irregular flow. An interlacing vascular network was seen. Some anastomoses were evident with the surrounding vascularization.

An anti-angiogenic treatment of 3 intravitreal ranimizumab injections and one aflibercept injection was administered PRN. We have been following this patient for 5 months now.

First Treatment, First Cycle

Seven Days after Injection: the fibrovascular area remained unchanged. Immediate important pruning of the thinner anastomoses and the loss of smaller vessels were observed. The network density decreased, with only some vessels highlighted. Residual flow was uneven. No feeder vessel could be seen.

Twenty-Eight Days after Injection: vessels and some anastomoses reappeared. The CNV mean area was smaller. There were fewer vessels with an increased caliber and increased flow.

A second treatment was performed at 34 days after the first treatment (second cycle).

2° Cycle – 7 Days after Injection: the fibrovascular area remained unchanged, and there was a decrease in the number of visible vessels.

2° Cycle – 42 Days after Injection: reproliferation of the vessels occurred, and they appeared similar to those that had collapsed. The fibrovascular area remained unchanged, and the vessel density was smaller. There were few vessels.

The third treatment was provided at 48 days after the second treatment.

The third cycle was similar to the first. The fibrovascular area remained unchanged. Visual acuity continued to improve over the 3 treatment cycles to 78 ETDRS letters (fig. 2).

After each new treatment, the same main vessels seemed to reappear, with increased flow and decreased branch density. Some main branches did not seem to be affected by the treatment. Some new sprouting occurred in new areas, and in other areas, small capillaries reopened. The fibrovascular area was constant, without any dimension variation.

Common Features of Cyclic Choroidal Neovascularization Early Evolution after Treatment

In our series, the early evolution of CNV after treatment exhibited common vascular features among the patients when examined by OCTA. We were able to add interesting new aspects of CNV morphology to current knowledge and observed anti-VEGF effects after only 24 h. Other authors have reported only a reduction in CNV size after anti-VEGF injection and feeder vessel preservation.

As reported in CNV type 1 neovascularization, anti-VEGF intravitreal injections promoted preservation of the central trunk vessels (feeder vessels) and a reduction of the entire circumferential anastomosis border [8] with a paucity of capillaries observed on OCTA. De Carlo et al. [7] de-

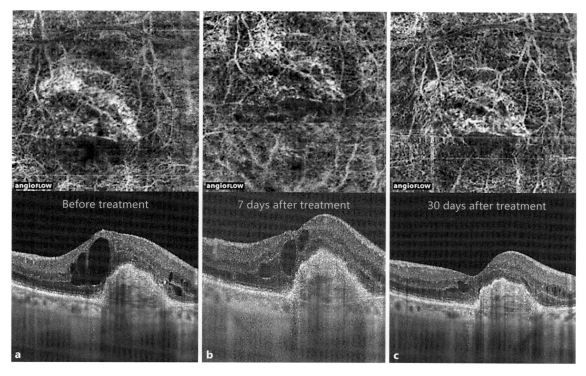

Fig. 2. First cycle after treatment of an 80-year-old man with naïve CNV in fibrovascular formation. **a** OCTA shows CNV in the left eye inside of a horizontal ovoid formation with a dark choriocapillaris ring-shaped area around the fibrotic formation. An irregular, fragmented neovascular network is seen inside of the fibrotic tissue. The vessels appear as a tangled network with small branches, a few vascular loops and irregular flow. An interlacing vascular network is seen. Some anastomoses are evident with the surrounding vascularization. **b** Seven days after injection: The fibrovascular area remains unchanged. The pruning of thinner anastomoses and the loss of smaller vessels are apparent. The network density is decreased, with only some vessels highlighted. Residual flow is uneven. No feeder vessel can be seen. **c** Twenty-eight days after injection: vessels and some anastomoses have reappeared. The CNV mean area is smaller. There are fewer vessels with increased caliber and flow.

scribed similar results, reporting that thirteen eyes with CNV showed consistent reductions in size after anti-VEGF injection. They also reported a case of apparent vessel perfusion detected on OCTA that did not show leakage on FA.

Kuehlewein et al. [9] also observed a progressive reduction in vascular lesions after intravitreal ranibizumab injection, with no change of the central large trunk. However, the OCTA intervals for the controls were too far from each other to follow the precise CNV evolution.

The vascular network remodeling observed in our patients with CNV neovascularization who received anti-VEGF injection shared similar characteristics with previously reported cases [7–9]. In addition, the anti-VEGF effects were observable after only 24 h.

Observations from Our Case Series

Our study has provided some important results regarding consistency in the patterns of cyclic CNV variations post-treatment in different patients. We observed changes that occurred over time, with alternating regression and progression phases. In fact, after administration of the injection, the pruning of smaller vessels was seen immediately, after only 24 h, with a reduction in the number of thinner anastomoses and the loss of thinner capillaries. The network density decreased, with only some major preexisting vessels highlighted. Residual flow was uneven and was more visible close to the afferent trunk. The results were as follows: an important loss of smaller vessels, microvascular rarefaction, and decreased vessel caliber, with vessel narrowing and apparent fragmentation. The decreases in the CNV area and vessel density were due to the loss of smaller capillaries. Smaller vessels were not visible due to collapse or to very slow flow. The vessel-related decreases lasted for 6–15 days.

Reopening or new sprouting of vessels was observable from 20 to 40 days after each injection. New vessel reproliferation and/or recanalization reappeared. The vessels at this stage looked grossly the same as those seen before treatment, but their diameters were greater. The average CNV area and vessel density were smaller. The remaining vessels showed increased calibers and increased flow around the afferent trunk.

Changes in the CNV diameter and area, number of capillaries and vessel sizes seemed to follow (after the loading phase) a cycle of 62.3 days in our series. After each cycle, the CNV had fewer visible branches and formed some anastomotic connections among larger vessels. Few capillaries were visualized within the lesions. The cycle was shorter during the loading phase, when the protocol indicates that inject should be performed after a 30-day interval.

Our observations on early CNV evolution seem to confirm observations by Spaide [8] in his series of late CNV evolution. Central trunk vessels are large in diameter given the relatively small lesion sizes, the vessels within the lesions show limited branching as they travel to the peripheral portions of the lesions, there are prominent anastomotic connections between large-diameter vessels, and variable amounts of peripheral anastomoses exist at the borders of many lesions. Spaide has stated that these observations do not preclude the possibility of capillaries being present, but not visualized, within the lesions. However, the salient characteristics reported by Spaide included large-diameter and prominent anastomoses of the vessels in treated CNV, as we observed in our own series.

Due to the high specificity of OCTA, it represents a better tool for obtaining detailed information on the course of CNV during anti-VEGF treatment. Furthermore, FA sometimes produces false positive results on CNV recurrence in the absence of active leakage.

In conclusion, OCTA is a useful noninvasive technique for investigating CNV morphology, features and activity, for which other methods can produce equivocal results.

Future studies using a larger sample size and examining different CNV types are necessary to support the potential clinical application of OCTA for CNV assessment and management.

Optical Coherence Tomography Angiography: Choroidal Neovascularization Type Determination and Follow-Up

OCTA allows for better recognition of the CNV type. OCTA images are reproducible and easy to generate, and the technique is noninvasive. There is no masking caused by dye leakage or pooling; thus, CNV pattern changes after therapy can be better evaluated.

In our series, all of the patients seemed to follow a 45–60-day cycle before the subsequent injection. After each injection, the pruning of smaller vessels was seen immediately (after 24 h), and this activity increased for 6–12 days until it reached a maximum level. This pruning was followed by the reopening or new sprouting of vessels 20–50 days later. The later cycles seemed to be longer. Our results on early CNV evolution seem to confirm the observations of Spaide on CNV abnormalization and arterialization. The pruning of small peripheral branches seems to strengthen the trunk. On OCTA, the closing of terminal vessels (anti-VEGF effects) seems to cause increased flow in the trunk after CNV reactivation.

Huang et al. [12] published a case in which they used frequent imaging to demonstrate a dramatic shutdown of CNV flow during the initial 2 weeks after antiangiogenic injection, followed by the reappearance of channels at 4 weeks and the reaccumulation of fluids at 6 weeks. To our knowledge, this is the first known short-interval dynamic analysis of the CNV treatment response using OCTA. Restoration of the CNV flow area may be a leading indicator of fluid reaccumulation and visual decline. The time course in this case suggests that OCTA scans performed every 14–15 days may be appropriate for determining the direction and rate of change in the CNV flow area and could provide information on whether extension of the treatment interval would be successful.

It is too early to affirm that OCTA can contribute important morphological data to aid in determining the timing of CNV treatment. More studies of a larger number of patients are needed to better understand early and late CNV evolution after treatment.

CNV feature alterations observed on OCTA will likely allow for determination of the optimal injection time if the PRN regimen is followed. Our small series contributes information regarding the characteristics of the early evolution of treated type 2 CNV. If our findings are confirmed, then OCTA may be considered useful for guiding the selection of the optimal interval between injections so that fluid reaccumulation does not occur. It is also intriguing to consider whether more frequent injections or the continuous depot delivery of an antiangiogenic medication that prevents the reappearance of CNV channels might affect CNV regression earlier and more permanently [12].

References

1 Owens SL: Indocyanine green angiography. Br J Ophthalmol 1996;80:263–266.
2 Do DV: Detection of new-onset choroidal neovascularization. Curr Opin Ophthalmol 2013;24:244–247.
3 Shah AR, Del Priore LV: Natural history of predominantly classic, minimally classic, and occult subgroups in exudative age-related macular degeneration. Ophthalmology 2009;116:1901–1907.
4 Wong TY, Chakravarthy U, Klein R, et al: The natural history and prognosis of neovascular age-related macular degeneration: a systematic review of the literature and meta-analysis. Ophthalmology 2008;115:116–126.
5 Jia Y, Tan O, Tokayer J, et al: Split-spectrum amplitude-decorrelation angiography with optical coherence tomography. Opt Express 2012;20:4710–4725.
6 Wei E, Jia Y, Tan O, et al: Parafoveal retinal vascular response to pattern visual stimulation assessed with OCT angiography. PLoS One 2013;8:e81343.
7 De Carlo TE, Bonini Filho MA, Chin AT, et al: Spectral-domain optical coherence tomography angiography of choroidal neovascularization. Ophthalmology 2015;122:1228–1238.
8 Spaide RF: Optical coherence tomography angiography signs of vascular abnormalization with antiangiogenic therapy for choroidal neovascularization. Am J Ophthalmol 2015;160:6–16.
9 Kuehlewein L, Sadda SR, Sarraf D: OCT angiography and sequential quantitative analysis of type 2 neovascularization after ranibizumab therapy. Eye (Lond) 2015;29:932–935.
10 Ferrara N: The role of vascular endothelial growth factor in pathological angiogenesis. Breast Cancer Res Treat 1995; 36:127–137.
11 Lumbroso B, Rispoli M, Savastano MC: Longitudinal optical coherence tomography – angiography study of type 2 naive choroidal neovascularization early response after treatment. Retina 2015; 35:2242–2251.
12 Huang D, Jia Y, Tan O, et al: Optical coherence tomography angiography of time course of choroidal neovascularization in response to anti-angiogenic treatment. Retina 2015;35:2260–2264.

Bruno Lumbroso
Centro Italiano Macula
Via Brofferio 7
IT–00195 Rome (Italy)
E-Mail bruno.lumbroso@gmail.com

Bandello F, Souied EH, Querques G (eds): OCT Angiography in Retinal and Macular Diseases.
Dev Ophthalmol. Basel, Karger, 2016, vol 56, pp 86–90 (DOI: 10.1159/000442783)

Optical Coherence Tomography Angiography of Fibrosis in Age-Related Macular Degeneration

Eric H. Souied[a] · Alexandra Miere[a] · Salomon Yves Cohen[a] · Oudy Semoun[a] · Giuseppe Querques[a, b]

[a]Department of Ophthalmology, Centre Hospitalier Intercommunal de Créteil, Universite Paris Est Créteil, Créteil, France;
[b]Department of Ophthalmology IRCCS San Raffaele Scientific Institute University Vita-Salute San Raffaele, Milan, Italy

Abstract

Purpose: To describe the optical coherence tomography angiography (OCTA) features of subretinal fibrosis in the context of exudative age-related macular degeneration. **Methods:** Patients diagnosed exudative age-related macular degeneration presenting with subretinal fibrosis were imaged by conventional multimodal imaging and OCTA. The patients were divided into the following two groups: group A, for eyes with active exudative features over the last 6 months, and group B, for eyes without any sign of exudation for >6 months. **Results:** In almost all of the patients, a high-flow network was detected inside of the fibrotic scar. We divided the vascular networks into the following three patterns: the pruned vascular tree, tangled network and vascular loop patterns. Furthermore, two types of low-flow structures, for which we coined the terms large flow void and dark halo, were observed. Both active and inactive lesions demonstrated the abovementioned patterns either individually or together. No difference was found between the two groups in the prevalent vascular network pattern of low-flow areas. **Conclusion:** OCTA of subretinal fibrosis revealed a perfused, abnormal vascular network, as well as collateral architectural changes in the outer retina and the choriocapillaris layer, in the majority of the studied eyes. These features are associated with both active and inactive fibrotic choroidal neovessels.

© 2016 S. Karger AG, Basel

Fibrosis and geographic atrophy are the end points of the natural history of neovascular age-related macular degeneration (AMD) [1]. Given the permanent structural damage to the retinal pigment epithelium and photoreceptors and the unlikelihood of improvement in visual acuity, few papers have assessed the subsequent tissue repair mechanisms that take place in both untreated and

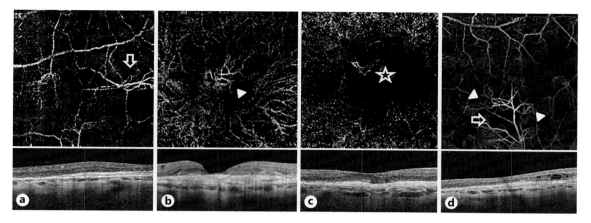

Fig. 1. Optical coherence tomographic angiography (OCTA) of exudative age-related macular degeneration (AMD) patients with subretinal fibrosis: neovascular patterns. **a** OCTA image delineates a vascular network in the outer retinal segments composed of large vessels with moderately high filamentous flow (white arrow) and no visible thinner capillaries. The corresponding B-scan shows a hyperreflective fibrous scar. **b** OCTA images of the outer retinal segments and corresponding B-scan showing the tangled neovascular network (arrowhead) as a high-flow structure composed of thin emerging branches and many collateral branches to the surrounding vessels. **c** OCTA images of the outer retinal segments and corresponding B-scan (**b**). **c** OCTA images of the outer retinal segments and corresponding B-scan reveal a high-flow, convoluted network (white star). **d** OCTA image and corresponding B-scan show a high-flow, central pruned vascular tree pattern (white arrow) combined with areas of tangled network (white arrowhead) in the terminal region. Adapted from Miere et al., Optical coherence tomography angiography features of subretinal fibrosis in age related macular degeneration. Retina, Nov 2015.

anti-vascular endothelial growth factor-treated eyes with subretinal fibrosis secondary to neovascular AMD [1, 2]. Furthermore, within the context of emerging new therapies (anti-platelet derived growth factor) [3] and technologies (optical coherence tomography angiography (OCTA)) [4], our study aims to provide a better understanding of the abnormal angiogenesis occurring in eyes with advanced neovascularization.

Multimodal imaging provides a comprehensive view of fibrosis. On color photographs, fibrosis is demonstrated by a well-delineated mound of white-yellowish tissue, corresponding to late staining and no leakage on fluorescein angiography [1]. On spectral-domain OCT, fibrosis appears as a compact, subretinal hyperreflective lesion, with variable degrees of loss of both the retinal pigment epithelium and ellipsoid zone [5]. Nevertheless, while the abovementioned imaging techniques provide details on the modified architectures of the retinal layers surrounding subretinal fibrosis, they do not provide specific information on structural changes that occur within the fibrotic scar itself. However, OCTA reveals key information on the status of the fibrous lesion, for example, the presence of a dormant or active neovascular network within the scar, giving rise to interesting imaging-pathologic correlations.

As a depth-resolved imaging technique [6, 7], OCTA is able to reveal, in almost all cases, a perfused vascular network within the fibrotic scar, together with collateral architectural changes in the outer retina and the choriocapillaris layer.

The following three major neovascular network patterns inside of fibrotic scars have been described in a recent study: the pruned vascular tree, tangled network, and vascular loop patterns [5]. Neovascular networks with the pruned vascular tree pattern (fig. 1a, 2) are composed of

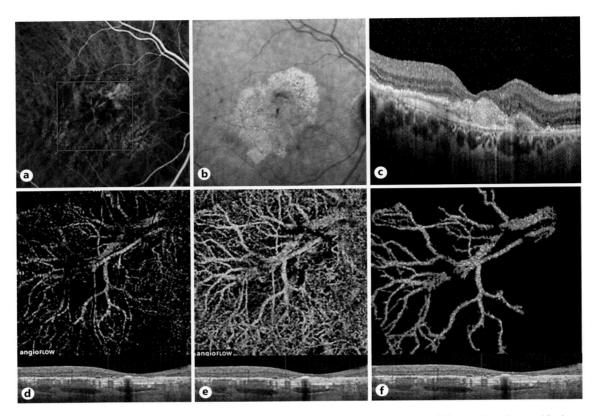

Fig. 2. Multimodal imaging of a 71-year-old patient with exudative AMD and subretinal fibrosis. Panels **a** and **b** show early- and late-phase indocyanine green angiography images, respectively. The red arrow in panel **a** indicates the central feeder vessel. Panel **c** shows the corresponding spectral-domain OCT image, revealing a hyperreflective, compact fibrotic lesion. In panel **d**, the OCTA image of the fibrous scar in the outer retinal segment is shown with the corresponding B-scan, revealing the pruned vascular tree pattern. Panel **e** shows the OCTA image of choriocapillaris segmentation with the corresponding B-scan, revealing a high-signal, eccentric lesion composed of important, moderately undulated vessels with few emergent collateral branches. Inside of the lesion, there is irregular flow. Panel **f** presents the subtracted, colorized neovascular network, as perceived in the segmentation corresponding to the whole fibrotic lesion.

important vessels with irregular flow, with no thinner capillaries visible when segmenting the fibrotic scar on OCTA. This pattern was present in half of the study eyes, either independently or together with another pattern. In all cases with the pruned vascular tree pattern, a central feeder vessel was detected (fig. 2). Likewise, the tangled network pattern (fig. 1b) is characterized by high flow and an interlacing vascular network, which is visible in the segmentation corresponding to the fibrous scar. The third high-flow pat-

tern is the vascular loop pattern (fig. 1c), which appears as a convoluted network on OCTA images. Additionally, the presence of two types of dark lesions, flow void and dark halo lesions, can be distinguished (fig. 3). The flow void lesion has a diffuse lack of signal in the segmentation corresponding to the fibrotic scar (fig. 3a) and was present in 63% of the eyes included in the study. The second type of dark area, the dark halo, surrounds the neovascular network and harbors a dark ring in the choriocapillaris seg-

Fig. 3. OCTA of exudative AMD patients with subretinal fibrosis: dark areas. **a** OCTA image of choriocapillaris segmentation and corresponding B-scan showing a large flow void as a diffuse lack of signal (dotted red line). **b** OCTA images of choriocapillaris segmentation and corresponding B-scan. A tangled neovascular network appears as a high-flow, round lesion composed of thin emerging branches. Note the dark area (green dotted line) surrounding the active choroidal neovascularization. Adapted from Miere et al. [5], Optical coherence tomography angiography features of subretinal fibrosis in age related macular degeneration. Retina, Nov 2015.

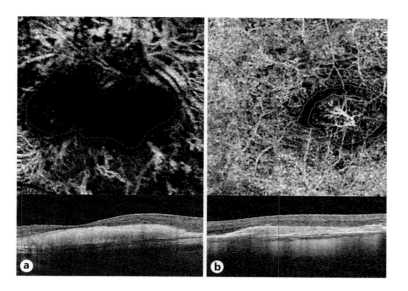

mentation (fig. 3b). This type of lesion appeared in 65% of the study eyes. The prevalence rates of the neovascular patterns were as follows: 53% for pruned vascular tree, 30% for tangled network and 48% for vascular loop, with no significant differences between the eyes with and without exudative features over the last 6 months.

These neovascular network patterns appear either independently or together (when there is a prevalent pattern within the lesion associated with elements from the other two patterns) (fig. 1d), generating the following two phenotypes of fibrotic lesions: the dead tree phenotype, including lesions with a main pruned vascular tree pattern, and the blossoming tree phenotype, for which the tangled network and vascular loop patterns prevail. We found highly significant associations between the vascular loop pattern and dark halo and between the flow void and dark halo. Moreover, the dead tree phenotype corresponds to irregular, filamentous flow [7] in networks formed by major vascular trunks (fig. 1, 3a), while the blossoming tree phenotype is rather curvy in shape and is correlated with high-flow

networks presenting with abundant anastomoses with the surrounding vascularization (fig. 1b–d, 3b). Spaide has explained that the higher flow observed in the remaining patent vessels could be due to a higher pressure differential and that this phenomenon is probably secondary to an increase in vascular resistance. Moreover, this increased flow in patent vessels would be a stimulus for arteriogenesis, which in consequence would result in generation of a larger vessel size [8].

OCTA discloses distinctive, abnormal vascular networks corresponding to fibrotic scars in the majority of cases that have been previously impossible to evaluate by fluorescein angiography or spectral-domain OCT alone. However, due to low visual acuity and lack of fixation, this technique is uninterpretable and/or time-consuming in some cases. Qualitative and quantitative assessments of these fibrotic neovascular lesions are interesting from both a pathogenic and clinical point of view – the likelihood of new exudative changes occurring within the neovascular lesion – thereby demonstrating the potential of OCTA as a standard technique for use in the assessment of neovascular AMD patients [5, 7–9].

References

1 Toth LA, Stevenson M, Chakravarthy U. Anti-vascular endothelial growth factor therapy for neovascular age-related macular degeneration: outcomes in eyes with poor initial vision. Retina 2015;35: 1957–1963.

2 Hwang JC, Del Priore LV, Freund KB, et al: Development of subretinal fibrosis after anti-VEGF treatment in neovascular age-related macular degeneration. Ophthalmic Surg Lasers Imaging 2011; 42:6–11.

3 Dugel PU, Kunimoto D, Quinlan E, et al: Anti-VEGF resistance in neovascular AMD: Role of PDGF antagonism. Paper presented at The Association for Research in Vision and Ophthalmology Annual Meeting, Denver, USA, May 2015.

4 Jia Y, Bailey ST, Wilson DJ, et al: Quantitative optical coherence tomography angiography of choroidal neovascularization in age-related macular degeneration. Ophthalmology 2014;121:1435–1444.

5 Miere A, Semoun O, Cohen SY, et al: Optical coherence tomography angiography features of subretinal fibrosis in age-related macular degeneration. Retina 2015;35:2275–2284.

6 Jia Y, Tan O, Tokayer J, et al: Split-spectrum amplitude-decorrelation angiography with optical coherence tomography. Opt Express 2012;20:4710–4725.

7 de Carlo TE, Bonini Filho MA, Chin AT, et al: Spectral-domain optical coherence tomography angiography of choroidal neovascularization. Ophthalmology 2015;122:1228–1238.

8 Spaide RF: Optical coherence tomography angiography signs of vascular abnormalization with antiangiogenic therapy for choroidal neovascularization. Am J Ophthalmol 2015;160:6–16.

9 Spaide RF, Klancnik JM Jr, Cooney MJ: Retinal vascular layers in macular telangiectasia type 2 imaged by optical coherence tomographic angiography. JAMA Ophthalmol 2015;133:66–73.

Eric H. Souied
Department of Ophthalmology, Centre Hospitalier Intercommunal de Créteil
Universite Paris Est Créteil, 40 Avenue de Verdun
FR–94000 Créteil (France)
E-Mail eric.souied@chicreteil.fr

Bandello F, Souied EH, Querques G (eds): OCT Angiography in Retinal and Macular Diseases.
Dev Ophthalmol. Basel, Karger, 2016, vol 56, pp 91–100 (DOI: 10.1159/000442784)

Optical Coherence Tomography Angiography of Dry Age-Related Macular Degeneration

Nadia K. Waheed[a] · Eric M. Moult[b] · James G. Fujimoto[b] · Philip J. Rosenfeld[c]

[a]New England Eye Center, Tufts University School of Medicine, Center, Boston, Mass., and [b]Department of Electrical Engineering and Computer Science and Research Laboratory of Electronics, Massachusetts Institute of Technology, Cambridge, Mass., and [c]Bascom Palmer Eye Institute, University of Miami Miller School of Medicine, Miami, Fla., USA

Abstract

Optical coherence tomography angiography (OCTA) can be used to visualize alterations in the choriocapillaris of patients with dry age-related macular degeneration (AMD). These changes seem to be present during all stages of the disease. Earlier stages are associated with patchy thinning of the choriocapillaris, while geographic atrophy is associated with loss of choriocapillaris lying under the area of geographic atrophy and asymmetric alteration of choriocapillaris at the margins of the geographic atrophy. The use of high-speed, long-wavelength swept-source OCT for angiography, with its better penetration into the choroid and high acquisition speeds, enable OCTA with scaled slowest detectable flow and fastest distinguishable flow. This will enable us to better investigate choriocapillaris changes in patients with dry AMD. The ability to image the choriocapillaris structure and flow impairments may be useful in the future for detecting and monitoring the progression of dry AMD and for monitoring treatment responses in clinical trials to therapies that target disease progression in dry AMD.

© 2016 S. Karger AG, Basel

Nonneovascular or dry age-related macular degeneration (AMD) is one of the leading causes of vision loss in people over 60 years of age in the developed world. Dry AMD accounts for 85–90% of all cases of AMD [1, 2]. In its early stages, it is characterized by the presence of drusen and pigmentary abnormalities resulting from alterations in the retinal pigment epithelium (RPE). In later stages, it can progress to geographic atrophy (GA) or outer retinal atrophy [3–6]. Late atrophic AMD is an important cause of irreversible vision loss, even in patients with neovascular AMD, because the use of vascular endothelial growth factor inhibitors successfully suppresses neovascularization and results in the progression of these lesions to atrophy [7].

Until recently, most research investigating AMD has been focused on the neovascular, or wet, form of AMD and the conversion from dry to wet AMD. While the pathological events leading from early-stage dry AMD to late-stage wet or atrophic AMD remain poorly understood, both histological and optical coherence tomography (OCT)-based studies have shown that the earliest detectable changes that characterize the progression of the disease occur at the interface of the retina and choroid, where the outer segments of the photoreceptors, RPE, Bruchs membrane, and choriocapillaris are located [8–12].

Early changes in AMD include the deposition of material within Bruchs membrane and between Bruchs membrane and the RPE. These deposits present clinically as a thickened sub-RPE layer, which includes drusen, and pigmentary abnormalities, which correspond to disruption of the RPE layer [13–16]. These changes are associated with progression down one of the following two late AMD pathways: the development of neovascularization or the development of atrophy, characterized by the loss of photoreceptors, the RPE, and the choriocapillaris.

A healthy RPE is essential for normal photoreceptor cell metabolism and the visual cycle. In dry AMD, RPE degeneration is accompanied by concomitant photoreceptor degeneration, giving rise to areas of GA [17]. However, the nature of the insults that initiate the pathway of RPE and subsequent photoreceptor cell loss have yet to be ascertained. Genetic factors, ischemia, inflammation and oxidative stress, RPE dysfunction, and the complement pathway all may play roles in the development of AMD [18–21]. However, there is considerable debate as to whether the initial changes take place in the choroid, in the RPE, or in the photoreceptors. There is evidence of early changes in the choroid, RPE, and photoreceptors in patients with dry AMD [22, 23].

OCT has been used extensively to study dry AMD. With the advent of high-resolution spectral-domain (SD) OCT, we have been able to observe and quantify the structural changes that occur in the retina and RPE and to some extent, the choroid, in patients with dry AMD. Drusen are evident as deposits in Bruchs membrane that elevate and distort the RPE, which appears to cause

outer retinal disruption and eventual breakdown of the RPE and photoreceptors. GA often follows the disappearance of drusen and is characterized by the well-delineated loss of the RPE, photoreceptors, and choriocapillaris [24]. Moreover, it has been demonstrated that there may be asymmetric changes in the outer retina at the margins of GA and that the locations of these changes in the photoreceptor outer segments surrounding the GA may predict the direction of GA progression [4]. Software enhancements in OCT have enabled the quantification of drusen volume and GA size [25].

Traditional intensity-based and ultra-high-resolution SD-OCT techniques provide images of anatomical details of the photoreceptors and RPE and show that structural changes precede the development of GA, but they do not provide detailed anatomic images of the choriocapillaris, which may be crucial for understanding the sequence of events that are responsible for disease progression. For example, a fundamental debate in AMD is whether it is a primary disease of the photoreceptors, the RPE, or the choriocapillaris or whether it results from the choreographed dysfunction among all three layers, with specific layers playing more dominant roles in different patients depending on their genetics, environment, and overall health. The incomplete picture of disease progression in AMD results in part from the need to extrapolate longitudinal changes derived from histopathological findings in autopsy eyes with AMD, which are obtained at fixed time points and leave unanswered questions about the progressive changes that result in end-stage disease. For example, we do not know whether photoreceptor loss is primarily due to an abnormality of the photoreceptors or whether RPE dysfunction leads to photoreceptor loss. If RPE dysfunction is the primary defect, then we need to determine whether RPE dysfunction is due to a primary RPE abnormality or whether it results from loss of the choriocapillaris. Up until now, we have been unable to untangle the web of interdependence between these three layers because we can only measure anatomic and functional changes in the photoreceptors *in vivo* and anatomic changes in the RPE *in vivo*, but we have been unable to visualize the microvasculature of the choriocapillaris *in vivo*. To help unravel the mystery of disease progression, we need to understand the temporal sequence of anatomic and functional changes in the macula. Optical coherence tomography angiography (OCTA) may bring clarity to the role of the choriocapillaris in disease progression. With the advent of OCTA, it is now also possible to visualize the vascular changes that occur in dry AMD [26–28].

OCTA provides three-dimensional, depth-resolved images of the vasculature in the retina and choroid. This enables us to independently evaluate the vasculature of the inner and outer retina and the choriocapillaris. Because the vascular images of OCTA are intrinsically co-registered with structural OCT data, it is possible to correlate the vascular changes with structural changes noted on OCT scans. Another advancement is the application of swept-source (SS) OCT technology to OCTA [29, 30]. SS-OCT technology has a lower sensitivity roll-off with depth and a longer wavelength, which enables better image penetration below the RPE and therefore better visualization of the choroid [31–33]. SS-OCT also can support faster A-scan acquisition rates compared with SD-OCT and provide greater retinal coverage. The faster acquisition speeds in SS-OCT are especially important because OCTA relies on decorrelation between sequentially acquired OCT B-scans of the eye [34, 35]; therefore, acquisition speed forces trade-offs among imaging time, retinal coverage and pixel density in OCTA data sets. Higher acquisition speeds also support OCTA protocols with multiple repeated B-scans and the use of techniques that can detect flow impairment, such as variable interscan time analysis (VISTA), which will be explained in greater detail below [36].

Early Age-Related Macular Degeneration

Early and intermediate AMD are characterized by drusen and pigmentary abnormalities, but it is unknown whether changes in the choriocapillaris occur at these stages. Drusen and RPE changes can be visualized on structural OCT images [17]. Software enhancements in SD-OCT instruments enable quantification of drusen volume and their progression over time [25]. With the advent of OCTA, it is now possible to visualize the microvasculature of the retina and choriocapillaris *in vivo* and to correlate microvascular alterations to structural changes in the retina and RPE [26, 27, 37].

As expected, no significant changes are present in the retinal vasculature in early AMD. However, OCTA of the choriocapillaris shows changes that may not be related to aging alone. OCTA imaging of the choriocapillaris in normal eyes shows a dense homogenous network, with a fine pattern in the macula that is near the transverse resolution limit of OCT imaging. More peripheral OCTA images of the choriocapillaris exhibit a lobular architecture, consistent with the known morphology reported by vascular casting studies. These patterns are observed using SD-OCT, centered at a wavelength of 840 nm, as well as using SS-OCT, centered at a longer wavelength of 1,050 nm. With age, the density of the choriocapillaris is likely to be reduced; however, a homogenous and regular pattern of vasculature is still present.

OCTA images of early non-neovascular AMD eyes suggest that there is a general reduction in choriocapillaris density compared to age-matched normal controls, with some focal areas of choriocapillaris loss or flow impairment. The dark patches at the level of the choriocapillaris that correspond to choriocapillaris loss may sometimes be accompanied by displacement of the larger choroidal vessels into the space previously occupied by the choriocapillaris. These changes become more marked in more severe cases. These findings are in agreement with histopathological studies, which have noted that drusen form over areas devoid of capillary lumens and extend into the intercapillary pillars [38, 39]. Increased drusen density in histopathologic studies has been shown to correspond to a decreased vascular density of the choriocapillaris [40]. Analysis of *en face* structural OCT-B images of early AMD has also shown a reduction in visible choriocapillaris compared with normal eyes, but with a reduction in the OCT signal intensity underlying the drusen, it can be challenging to distinguish between loss of signal and loss of the choriocapillaris [22].

Although these changes in choriocapillaris density are visible in both SD-OCT and SS-OCT images, SS-OCT systems have better penetration into the choroid and therefore enable more reliable visualization of the choriocapillaris. In SD-OCT systems, drusen and RPE changes are more likely to cause signal attenuation shadowing. Strong structural OCT signals are required to obtain OCTA images, and shadowing causes dark areas on *en face* OCTA at the level of the choriocapillaris that are caused by poor signal rather than lack of blood flow. These areas of shadowing (as opposed to decreased perfusion) can be identified by concurrently looking at an *en face* OCT intensity image at the level of the choriocapillaris and an OCTA image and by examining a cross-sectional OCT image of the area of suspected choriocapillaris pathology. Areas of shadowing will appear dark on both the OCT intensity image and the angiographic image, whereas areas of decreased blood flow will appear normal on the intensity image but will appear dark on the *en face* OCTA image. Areas of shadowing are much more prevalent in SD-OCT images than in SS-OCT images because longer wavelengths have increased image penetration; thus, it is much easier to assess loss of choriocapillaris flow on SS-OCTA images than on SD-OCTA images. Figure 1 shows a composite image of same-day SS-OCTA and the corresponding *en face* OCT intensity images at the level of the choriocapillaris (fig. 1b, c), an SD-OCTA image with the corresponding *en face* OCT intensity image at the level of the choriocapillaris (fig. 1e, f) and the corresponding B-scan (fig. 1d) and a same-day color fundus image. The green arrows show an area of shadowing under the drusen, visible as a dark area on both the intensity and angiographic images. Note that the SS-OCTA image at the 840 nm wavelength (fig. 1b) has less pronounced shadowing in the area underneath the drusen than the SD-OCTA image (fig. 1e) at 1,050 nm due to the lower attenuation experienced by longer wavelengths.

Late Dry Age-Related Macular Degeneration

In patients with GA, OCTA shows loss of choriocapillaris flow under the regions of GA. In these areas of choriocapillaris alteration, larger choroidal vessels may be displaced into the area ordinarily occupied by the choriocapillaris and may be seen on the *en face* OCTA image at the depth level where the choriocapillaris is ordinarily seen. Figure 2 shows SS-OCTA images from a patient with GA, with corresponding red-free (fig. 2a) and fundus autofluorescence images (fig. 2b). In this patient, there were no changes in the retinal vasculature, as visible on OCTA segmented at the level of the retinal vasculature in figure 2c. In many cases, the areas of choriocapillaris alterations extend beyond the margins of GA in an asymmetric pattern (fig. 2d, e). These alterations outside of the margins of GA may be quite extensive or may be very limited and subtle. In a smaller number of cases, the choriocapillaris alterations may be limited to the area of GA and may not extend beyond that area. The changes underlying the area of GA are usually well visualized on both SD- and SS-OCTA since the RPE in these areas is missing and therefore does not attenuate the SD-OCT signal. However, especially at the margins of GA where the RPE is still intact, it may be more difficult to visualize changes in the choriocapillaris with SD-OCT.

One of the debates regarding visualization of choriocapillaris alterations in patients with GA

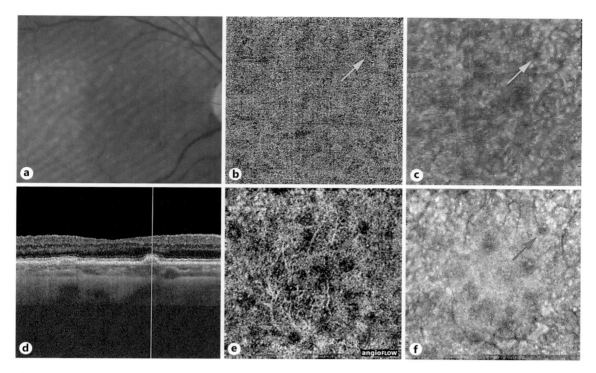

Fig. 1. A composite image of a color photo (**a**) and a same-day swept-source optical coherence tomography (OCT) angiography (OCTA) image and the corresponding *en face* OCT intensity image at the level of the choriocapillaris (CC) (**b, c**) and a spectral-domain OCTA image with the corresponding *en face* OCT intensity image at the level of the CC (**e, f**) and the corresponding B-scan (**d**). The green arrows show an area of shadowing under drusen, visible as a dark area on both the intensity and angiographic images. Note that the swept-source OCTA (**b**) image has less pronounced shadowing in the area underneath the drusen than the spectral-domain OCTA image (**e**), likely to due to improved choroidal penetration at longer wavelengths. The corresponding OCTA image (**b**) shows a relatively normal CC with little, if any, dropout of the CC.

Fig. 2. Fundus autofluorescence, OCT and OCTA in a 75-year-old patient with nonexudative age-related macular degeneration with geographic atrophy (GA). The fundus autofluorescence (**a**) and mean *en face* projection of the entire OCT volume (**b**) clearly show the region of GA, outlined by the yellow dashed contour (**b**). The GA region appears lighter due to increased light penetration into the choroid caused by retinal pigment epithelium atrophy. **c** The mean *en face* projection of the OCTA volume through the depths spanned by the retinal vasculature; the vasculature appears normal. (**d**) A 4.4-μm-thick *en face* OCTA slab at the CC level obtained using a 1.5-ms interscan time. The yellow dashed contour from (**b**) is superimposed, and a severe CC alteration appears within it. The severe CC alteration is also evident outside of the GA margin. (**e**) The same 4.4-μm-thick *en face* OCTA CC slab as (**d**), obtained using a 3.0-ms interscan time. Note how some areas with a low decorrelation signal (**d**) have increased decorrelation (**e**), suggesting flow impairment rather than complete atrophy. Enlarged views of the solid orange and green boxes (**d, e**) are shown (**f, g**), respectively. Note that some choroidal vessels that are not visible (**f**) become visible (**g**). Enlarged views of the dashed orange and green boxes (**d, e**) are shown (**h, i**), respectively. Note that some of the regions with low decorrelation signals (**h**) have higher decorrelation signals (**i**), suggesting flow impairment along the GA margin. OCT (top) and OCTA (bottom) B-scans through the red, blue, and purple horizontal dashed lines (**d**) are shown (**j–l**), respectively. All scale bars are 1 mm. *(For figure see next page.)*

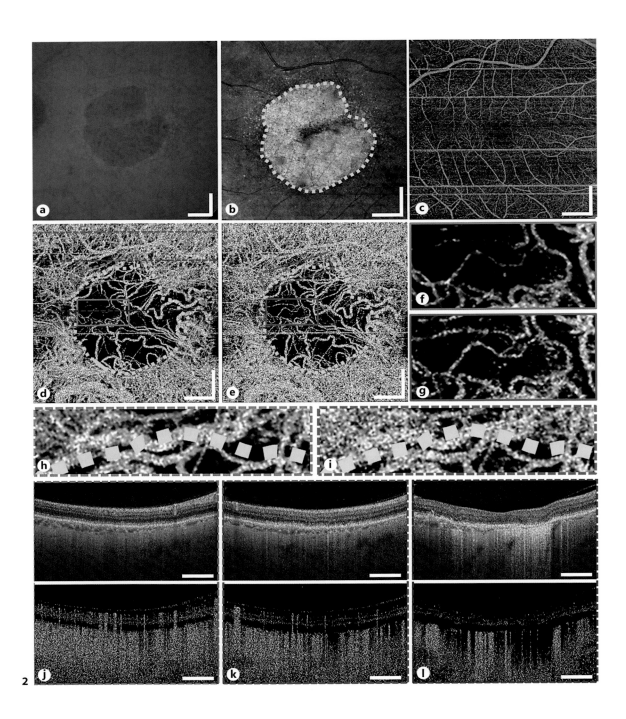

is whether they truly represent the absence of flow or merely reduced flow. OCTA creates flow images by comparing differences between consecutive OCT B-scan images. Micro-saccadic eye motion is always present, and changes due to erythrocyte flow must be separated from overall retinal motion. If the velocity of flow in the vessels is very slow, then OCTA may not be able to detect this slow flow versus the parasitic retinal motion. In addition, if flow is fast, then the OCTA image saturates (fast flow appears white), and variations in flow cannot be differentiated.

Thus, OCTA machines have a slowest detectable flow, or sensitivity threshold, below which they cannot detect flow at slow speeds, as well as a fastest distinguishable flow, or saturation limit, above which different flow speeds appear the same. The slowest detectable flow depends on the time between repeated B-scans, with longer interscan times producing a lower slowest detectable flow rate because erythrocytes have more time to move between B-scans. In addition, a longer interscan time also reduces the fastest distinguishable flow rate. The interscan time of current SD-OCT machines is 5 ms, while that of the SS-OCTA prototype instrument reported here is 1.5 ms. SD-OCT and SS-OCT instruments have acquisition speeds of 70,000 and 400,000 A-scans per second, respectively. The faster scanning speed allows SS-OCT to acquire larger numbers of repeated B-scans for the OCTA scanning protocol in the same amount of time as SD-OCT. This allows OCTA data to be generated between B-scans with longer versus shorter interscan times. Viewing the same areas on consecutive B-scans (fig. 2d) versus every second B-scan (fig. 2e) using OCTA helps to identify areas of flow impairment that may not be distinguishable using instruments with slower acquisition speeds or OCTA with long interscan times. Using SS-OCTA with VISTA to vary the slowest detectable flow and fastest discernable flow rates, we can show that choriocapillaris alterations within the borders of GA tend to have slow flow rates and may be primarily atrophic, while choriocapillaris alterations beyond the borders of GA have flow impairment. Figure 2f and g show magnified images that correspond to a region within the borders of GA analyzed using OCTA with varying interscan times. In figure 2g, we are better able to visualize slow flow in some vessels in this region of atrophy. However, compared to the surrounding choriocapillaris, it is clear that there are considerable areas of absent flow or reduced flow underlying this area of GA. The images shown in figure 2h and i correspond to a region at the margin of GA analyzed using varying interscan times. Figure 2h shows an OCTA image obtained with a 1.5-ms interscan time, while figure 2i depicts an image acquired with a 3.0-ms interscan time. With in-

Fig. 3. Variable interscan time analysis. OCTA images are generated using 5 repeated B-scans at the same location, with a time interval of 1.5 ms between each scan. Comparisons between B-scans are used to generate the decorrelation signal. Decorrelation signals can be generated by comparing adjacent B-scans, with an interscan time of 1.5 ms (**a**), or between every second B-scan, increasing the interscan time to 3 ms (**d**). Figures (**b**, **e**) show schematic representations of how the decorrelation signal varies with the erythrocyte flow speed. Areas with no flow generate a decorrelation signal that appears black, while areas with high flow appear as white on OCTA. The dynamic range of OCTA for each interscan time is marked with brackets, indicating the slowest detectable flow and the fastest distinguishable flow. The asterisk, square, and circle indicate three hypothetical flow speeds. The slow flow, marked with the asterisk, does not fall within the OCTA dynamic range with the 1.5-ms interscan time, and it cannot be seen on the corresponding OCTA (**c**). However, when the interscan time is increased to 3 ms, this slow flow can be visualized. When the interscan time is increased to 3 ms, many vessels are visible that are either partially visible or absent on OCTA with an interscan time of 1.5 ms (**d**). Conversely, comparing OCTA with a 3.0-ms interscan time to OCTA with a 1.5-ms interscan time identifies area of flow impairment that are not distinguishable on the image obtained with a 3.0-ms interscan time alone. The scale bars are 250 μm, and the images are enlarged views from a 6 × 6 mm field of view.

(For figure see next page.)

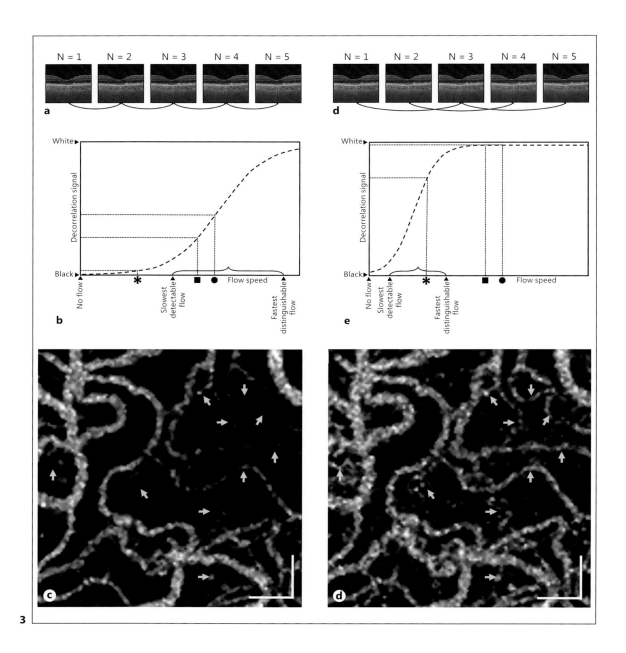

Figure 3

creased interscan times, we are able to better visualize that most of the areas of choriocapillaris alteration in this region have slow flow rather than the complete loss of flow. Conversely, if OCTA was performed using only a longer interscan time (which would be typical for SD-OCT instruments), then it would not be possible to distinguish areas of flow impairment.

It is still unclear why these choriocapillaris flow changes take place in patients with GA. However, these changes clearly seem to precede the obvious detectable atrophic structural changes in the RPEs and retinas of these patients observed using conventional structural OCT. These results suggest that microstructural changes detectable on OCTA are present before they become detectable on conventional intensity-based OCT. Additional longitudinal studies are needed to better characterize the progression of these choriocapillaris alterations. In response to the debate about whether the primary site of pathogenesis of GA is the choriocapillaris or the RPE, these OCTA findings that choriocapillaris alterations appear to be at least the size of GA, and often greater, appear to support the hypothesis that choriocapillaris loss may precede RPE changes. However, additional studies using high-resolution SD-OCT may be needed to confirm these findings.

In summary, OCTA can be used to visualize alterations in the choriocapillaris of patients with dry AMD. These changes seem to be present during all stages of the disease. The use of high-speed, long-wavelength SS-OCT for angiography, with its better penetration into the choroid and high acquisition speeds, enable OCTA with VISTA to be performed. Scaling the slowest detectable flow and fastest distinguishable flow will enable us to better investigate choriocapillaris changes in patients with dry AMD. The ability to image the choriocapillaris structure and flow impairments may be useful in the future for detecting and monitoring the progression of dry AMD and for monitoring treatment responses in clinical trials to therapies that target disease progression in dry AMD.

References

1 Velez-Montoya R, Oliver SC, Olson JL, Fine SL, Quiroz-Mercado H, Mandava N: Current knowledge and trends in age-related macular degeneration: genetics, epidemiology, and prevention. Retina 2014;34:423–441.

2 Friedman DS, OColmain BJ, Munoz B, Tomany SC, McCarty C, de Jong PT, et al: Prevalence of age-related macular degeneration in the United States. Arch Ophthalmol 2004;122:564–572.

3 Fleckenstein M, Schmitz-Valckenberg S, Adrion C, Kramer I, Eter N, Helb HM, et al: Tracking progression with spectral-domain optical coherence tomography in geographic atrophy caused by age-related macular degeneration. Invest Ophthalmol Vis Sci 2010;51:3846–3852.

4 Nunes RP, Gregori G, Yehoshua Z, Stetson PF, Feuer W, Moshfeghi AA, et al: Predicting the progression of geographic atrophy in age-related macular degeneration with SD-OCT en face imaging of the outer retina. Ophthalmic Surg Lasers Imaging Retina 2013;44:344–359.

5 Klein R, Klein BE, Linton KL: Prevalence of age-related maculopathy. The Beaver Dam Eye Study. Ophthalmology 1992; 99:933–943.

6 Ferris FL 3rd, Wilkinson CP, Bird A, Chakravarthy U, Chew E, Csaky K, et al: Clinical classification of age-related macular degeneration. Ophthalmology 2013;120:844–851.

7 Velez-Montoya R, Oliver SC, Olson JL, Fine SL, Mandava N, Quiroz-Mercado H: Current knowledge and trends in age-related macular degeneration: todays and future treatments. Retina 2013; 33:1487–1502.

8 Complications of Age-related Macular Degeneration Prevention Trial Research Group: Risk factors for choroidal neovascularization and geographic atrophy in the complications of age-related macular degeneration prevention trial. Ophthalmology 2008;115:1474–1479, 9.e1–e6.

9 Joachim N, Mitchell P, Rochtchina E, Tan AG, Wang JJ: Incidence and progression of reticular drusen in age-related macular degeneration: findings from an older Australian cohort. Ophthalmology 2014;121:917–925.

10 Joachim ND, Mitchell P, Kifley A, Wang JJ: Incidence, progression, and associated risk factors of medium drusen in age-related macular degeneration: findings from the 15-Year follow-up of an Australian Cohort. JAMA Ophthalmol 2015;133:698–705.

11 Schuman SG, Koreishi AF, Farsiu S, Jung SH, Izatt JA, Toth CA: Photoreceptor layer thinning over drusen in eyes with age-related macular degeneration imaged in vivo with spectral-domain optical coherence tomography. Ophthalmology 2009;116:488–496.e2.

12 Moussa K, Lee JY, Stinnett SS, Jaffe GJ: Spectral domain optical coherence tomography-determined morphologic predictors of age-related macular degeneration-associated geographic atrophy progression. Retina 2013;33:1590–1599.

13 Lutty G, Grunwald J, Majji AB, Uyama M, Yoneya S: Changes in choriocapillaris and retinal pigment epithelium in age-related macular degeneration. Mol Vis 1999;5:35.

14 Curcio CA, Millican CL: Basal linear deposit and large drusen are specific for early age-related maculopathy. Arch Ophthalmol 1999;117:329–339.

15 Curcio CA, Messinger JD, Sloan KR, McGwin G, Medeiros NE, Spaide RF: Subretinal drusenoid deposits in nonneovascular age-related macular degeneration: morphology, prevalence, topography, and biogenesis model. Retina 2013;33:265–276.

16 Zhang Y, Wang X, Rivero EB, Clark ME, Witherspoon CD, Spaide RF, et al: Photoreceptor perturbation around subretinal drusenoid deposits as revealed by adaptive optics scanning laser ophthalmoscopy. Am J Ophthalmol 2014;158: 584–596.e1.

17 Bhutto I, Lutty G: Understanding Age-related Macular Degeneration (AMD): relationships between the photoreceptor/retinal pigment epithelium/Bruchs membrane/choriocapillaris complex. Mol Aspects Med 2012;33:295–317.

18 Curcio CA, Johnson M, Huang JD, Rudolf M: Aging, age-related macular degeneration, and the response-to-retention of apolipoprotein B-containing lipoproteins. Prog Retin Eye Res 2009; 28:393–422.

19 Seddon JM, Reynolds R, Yu Y, Daly MJ, Rosner B: Risk models for progression to advanced age-related macular degeneration using demographic, environmental, genetic, and ocular factors. Ophthalmology 2011;118:2203–2211.

20 Age-Related Eye Disease Study Research Group: Risk factors for the incidence of advanced age-related macular degeneration in the Age-Related Eye Disease Study (AREDS) AREDS report no. 19. Ophthalmology 2005;112:533–539.

21 Seddon JM, Francis PJ, George S, Schultz DW, Rosner B, Klein ML: Association of CFH Y402H and LOC387715 A69S with progression of age-related macular degeneration. JAMA 2007;297:1793–1800.

22 Sohrab M, Wu K, Fawzi AA: A pilot study of morphometric analysis of choroidal vasculature in vivo, using en face optical coherence tomography. PLoS One 2012;7:e48631.

23 McLeod DS, Grebe R, Bhutto I, Merges C, Baba T, Lutty GA: Relationship between RPE and choriocapillaris in age-related macular degeneration. Invest Ophthalmol Vis Sci 2009;50:4982–4991.

24 Wu Z, Luu CD, Ayton LN, Goh JK, Lucci LM, Hubbard WC, et al: Optical coherence tomography-defined changes preceding the development of drusen-associated atrophy in age-related macular degeneration. Ophthalmology 2014;121: 2415–2422.

25 Freeman SR, Kozak I, Cheng L, Bartsch DU, Mojana F, Nigam N, et al: Optical coherence tomography-raster scanning and manual segmentation in determining drusen volume in age-related macular degeneration. Retina 2010;30:431–435.

26 de Carlo TE, Romano A, Waheed N, Duker JS: A review of Optical Coherence Tomography Angiography (OCTA). International Journal of Retina and Vitreous 2015;1:5.

27 Matsunaga D, Yi J, Puliafito CA, Kashani AH: OCT angiography in healthy human subjects. Ophthalmic Surg Lasers Imaging Retina 2014;45:510–515.

28 Jia Y, Bailey ST, Hwang TS, McClintic SM, Gao SS, Pennesi ME, et al: Quantitative optical coherence tomography angiography of vascular abnormalities in the living human eye. Proc Natl Acad Sci U S A 2015;112:E2395–E2402.

29 Moult E, Choi W, Waheed NK, Adhi M, Lee B, Lu CD, et al: Ultrahigh-speed swept-source OCT angiography in exudative AMD. Ophthalmic Surg Lasers Imaging Retina 2014;45:496–505.

30 Choi W, Mohler KJ, Potsaid B, Lu CD, Liu JJ, Jayaraman V, et al: Choriocapillaris and choroidal microvasculature imaging with ultrahigh speed OCT angiography. PLoS ONE 2013;8:e81499.

31 Unterhuber A, Povazay B, Hermann B, Sattmann H, Chavez-Pirson A, Drexler W: In vivo retinal optical coherence tomography at 1,040 nm – enhanced penetration into the choroid. Opt Express 2005;13:3252–3258.

32 Povazay B, Hermann B, Unterhuber A, Hofer B, Sattmann H, Zeiler F, et al: Three-dimensional optical coherence tomography at 1,050 versus 800 nm in retinal pathologies: enhanced performance and choroidal penetration in cataract patients. J Biomed Opt 2007;12: 041211.

33 Adhi M, Liu JJ, Qavi AH, Grulkowski I, Lu CD, Mohler KJ, et al: Choroidal analysis in healthy eyes using swept-source optical coherence tomography compared to spectral domain optical coherence tomography. Am J Ophthalmol 2014;157:1272–1281.e1.

34 Jia Y, Tan O, Tokayer J, Potsaid B, Wang Y, Liu JJ, et al: Split-spectrum amplitude-decorrelation angiography with optical coherence tomography. Opt Express 2012;20:4710–4725.

35 Tokayer J, Jia Y, Dhalla AH, Huang D: Blood flow velocity quantification using split-spectrum amplitude-decorrelation angiography with optical coherence tomography. Biomed Opt Express 2013;4: 1909–1924.

36 Kraus MF, Potsaid B, Mayer MA, Bock R, Baumann B, Liu JJ, et al: Motion correction in optical coherence tomography volumes on a per A-scan basis using orthogonal scan patterns. Biomed Opt Express 2012;3:1182–1199.

37 Nagiel A, Sadda SR, Sarraf D: A promising future for optical coherence tomography angiography. JAMA Ophthalmol 2015;133:629–630.

38 Lengyel I, Tufail A, Hosaini HA, Luthert P, Bird AC, Jeffery G: Association of drusen deposition with choroidal intercapillary pillars in the aging human eye. Invest Ophthalmol Vis Sci 2004;45: 2886–2892.

39 Sarks SH, Arnold JJ, Killingsworth MC, Sarks JP: Early drusen formation in the normal and aging eye and their relation to age related maculopathy: a clinicopathological study. Br J Ophthalmol 1999;83:358–368.

40 Mullins RF, Johnson MN, Faidley EA, Skeie JM, Huang J: Choriocapillaris vascular dropout related to density of drusen in human eyes with early age-related macular degeneration. Invest Ophthalmol Vis Sci 2011;52:1606–1612.

Philip J. Rosenfeld, MD, PhD, Professor of Ophthalmology
Bascom Palmer Eye Institute
900 NW 17th St.
Miami, FL 33136 (USA)
E-Mail prosenfeld@med.miami.edu

Bandello F, Souied EH, Querques G (eds): OCT Angiography in Retinal and Macular Diseases.
Dev Ophthalmol. Basel, Karger, 2016, vol 56, pp 101–106 (DOI: 10.1159/000442800)

Optical Coherence Tomography Angiography of Choroidal Neovascularization Secondary to Pathologic Myopia

Giuseppe Querques[a, b] · Federico Corvi[a] · Lea Querques[a] · Eric H. Souied[b] ·
Francesco Bandello[a]

[a]Department of Ophthalmology IRCCS San Raffaele Scientific Institute University Vita-Salute San Raffaele, Milan, Italy;
[b]Department of Ophthalmology, Centre Hospitalier Intercommunal de Créteil, Paris Est University, Créteil, France

Abstract

Purpose: To analyze the ability of optical coherence tomography angiography (OCT-A) to detect the presence of myopic choroidal neovascularization (CNV) and to describe structural features of myopic CNV on OCT-A. **Methods:** Patients with CNV secondary to high myopia (>6 diopters and >26 mm axial length) underwent multimodal imaging, including multicolor imaging, fluorescein angiography, spectral-domain (SD)-OCT and OCT-A. The OCT-A features of CNV were analyzed and correlated with the angiography and SD-OCT findings. **Results:** On OCTA, the CNV appeared as a large hyperintense vascular anastomotic network at the edge of the lesion. On the basis of the OCT-A images and reports in the literature, we propose the following two terms for describing myopic CNV characteristics: 'interlacing' and 'tangled' vascular networks. **Conclusion:** OCT-A is a very useful tool for the diagnosis and evaluation of CNV complicating high myopia; however, it does not appear to be sufficient when used alone and should be considered for use in combination with SD-OCT and conventional angiography.   © 2016 S. Karger AG, Basel

High myopia is defined by an axial length of the eye of greater than 26 mm and by a refractive error of –6 diopters or more. Eyes with a high axial length are described as having pathologic myopia when they manifest degenerative changes of the sclera, choroid, and retina [1]. In pathologic myopia, progressive posterior segment elongation and deformation may lead to the development of macular lesions, such as myopic choroidal neovascularization (CNV) [2]. The recommended diagnostic examinations are fundus biomicros-

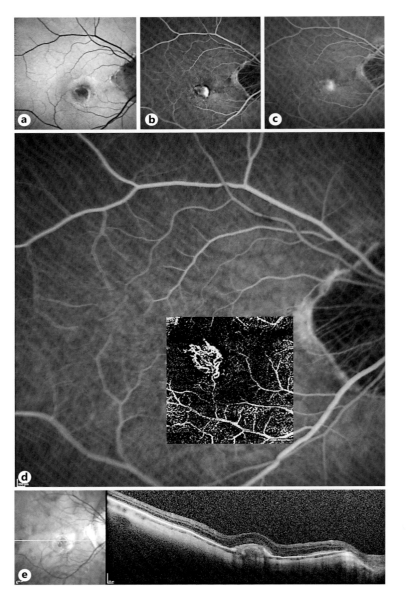

Fig. 1. Multimodal imaging of the right eye of a 56-year-old male with active myopic choroidal neovascularization (CNV). **a** Blue fundus autofluorescence shows a hypofluorescent area surrounded by a hyperfluorescent ring. **b** Early-phase fluorescein angiography (FA) reveals a hyperfluorescent area, with leakage during the late phase (**c**), surrounded by a hypofluorescent ring, suggestive of type 2 (classic) active CNV. **d** *En face* optical coherence tomography angiography (OCT-A) section (3 × 3 mm) just below the retinal pigment epithelium shows a dense, interlacing type 2 neovascular network with a well-circumscribed appearance. **e** Spectral-domain OCT B-scan reveals a hyperreflective lesion with shallow subretinal hyporeflective fluid suggestive of active type 2 CNV.

copy, fluorescein angiography (FA) and spectral-domain optical coherence tomography (SD-OCT) [3]. Myopic CNV present typically as 'classic' or 'type 2' on FA, with well-defined hyperfluorescence on early frames and leakage of the dye on late frames. SD-OCT shows a hyperreflective lesion located beneath the neurosensory retina, often associated with discrete retinal changes, including edema and neurosensory serous retinal detachment. The combination of SD-OCT and FA has been demonstrated to be more sensitive than FA alone or SD-OCT alone [4–6]. Optical coherence tomography angiography (OCT-A) is a novel and noninvasive imaging tool

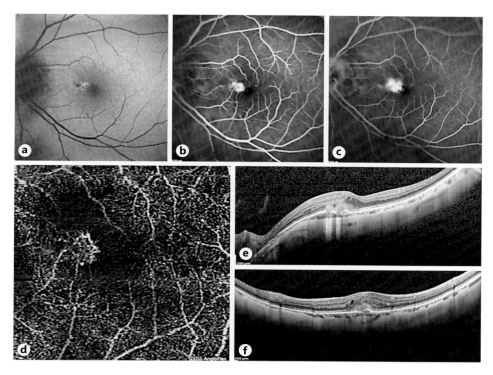

Fig. 2. Multimodal imaging of the left eye of a 51-year-old female with active myopic CNV. **a** Blue fundus autofluorescence reveals a hypofluorescent area surrounded by a hyperfluorescent ring. **b** Early-phase FA reveals a hyperfluorescent area, with leakage during the late phase (**c**) surrounded by a hypofluorescent ring, suggestive of type 2 (classic) active CNV. **d** *En face* OCT-A section (3 × 3 mm) just below retinal pigment epithelium shows a dense interlacing type 2 neovascular network with a well-circumscribed appearance. **e, f** Spectral-domain OCT B-scans show a hyper-reflective lesion with a small amount of subretinal hyporeflective fluid, suggestive of active type 2 CNV.

and *en face* technique that provides 3D images of dynamic blood perfusion within microcirculatory tissue beds. The imaging contrast of optical microangiography images is based on the intrinsic optical scattering of signals backscattered by the moving of blood cells in patent blood vessels [7].

Here, we report the abilities of phase-based (Doppler shift or variance) and intensity-based (speckle variance, decorrelation, and frequency filtering) OCT-A (AngioPlex™, CIRRUS HD-OCT model 5000, Carl Zeiss Meditec, Inc., Dublin, USA) to detect the presence of myopic CNV and to identify the morphological features of active or inactive CNV.

On OCT-A, myopic CNV appears as a large hyperintense vascular anastomotic network. On the basis of its characteristics on OCT-A, we propose that the following two types of myopic CNV exist: 'interlacing' and 'tangled' vascular networks [8, 9]. The interlacing network is characterized by dense vascular hyperintensity with a well-circumscribed appearance on OCT-A. This appearance is often associated with neovascular activity on conventional imaging, including FA and OCT B-scanning (fig. 1–3). The tangled network is defined by a loosely laced appearance on OCT-A. This appearance is often associated with the absence of neovascular activity on conven-

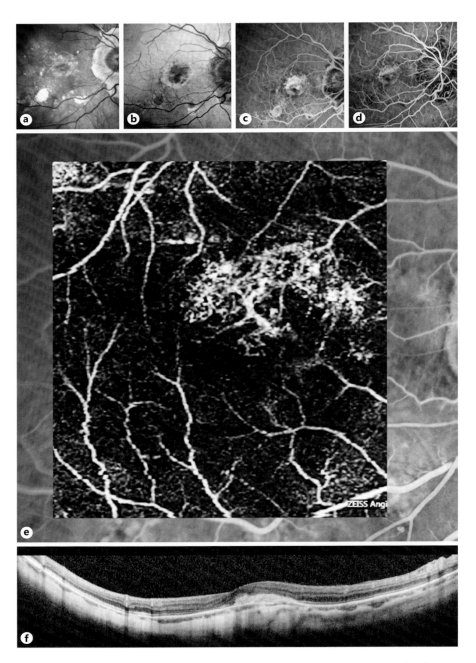

Fig. 3. Multimodal imaging of the right eye of a 62-year-old female affected with active myopic CNV. **a** Blue fundus autofluorescence and (**b**) multicolor images show white areas of focal chorioretinal atrophy with macular hemorrhage. **c** Early-phase FA reveals a hyperfluorescent area, with leakage during the late phase (**d**) surrounded by a hypofluorescent ring, suggestive of type 2 (classic) active CNV. **e** *En face* OCT-A section (3 × 3 mm) from just below the retinal pigment epithelium shows a dense interlacing type 2 neovascular network with a well-circumscribed appearance. **f** Spectral-domain OCT B-scan shows a hyper-reflective lesion with a small amount of subretinal hyporeflective fluid, suggestive of active type 2 CNV.

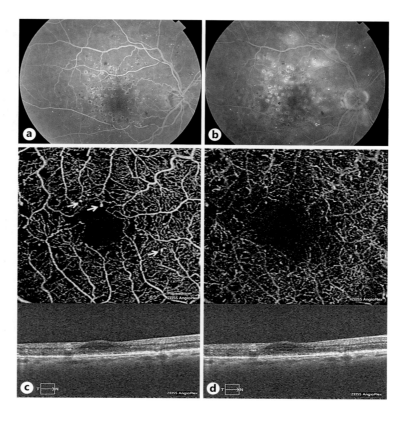

Fig. 2. FA, OCTA and OCT of a patient with nonproliferative diabetic retinopathy. **a, b** Early- and late-phase FA images reveal microaneurysms as outpouchings of the arteriolar wall with leakage. **c** Three-by-three millimeter OCT angiogram of the superficial capillary plexus and corresponding OCT B-scan. OCTA image, showing an enlarged FAZ, multiple microaneurysms (arrows) and capillary nonperfusion areas that are much more apparent in the deep capillary plexus. **d** Three-by-three millimeter OCT angiogram of the deep capillary plexus and corresponding OCT B-scan, showing remodeling of the FAZ, which looks even more enlarged compared to the superficial capillary plexus.

normalities and retinal neovascularization. Since fluorescein is partially unbound in the bloodstream, it can leak out of incompetent blood vessels. Visualization of the leakage of fluorescein dye over time is useful for showing breakdown of the blood-retinal barrier. This is best exemplified in diabetic macular edema: FA shows diffuse late hyperfluorescence due to leakage, which may assume a flower-petal pattern if cystoid macular edema is present. In eyes with PDR, retinal or optic disc neovascularization is also characterized by intensive fluorescein leakage.

Although FA can provide accurate information on retinal vasculopathy, better detection of peripheral neovascularization and the extent of retinal nonperfusion has been obtained using ultra-wide-field FA. Compared with standard field FA, this diagnostic imaging modality may reveal more pathological changes, such as early signs that might otherwise have been missed and that may suggest greater disease severity [10].

Although both standard FA and ultra-wide-field FA are very clinically useful, they have some limitations. They are invasive techniques in which a fluorescent dye is injected into the bloodstream, with the risk of severe adverse effects, including anaphylaxis and death, although such adverse effects are extremely rare. In addition, they do not contribute much to the evaluation of retinal morphology and its thickness profile, and visualization of the deep retinal and choroidal vessels is limited.

Optical Coherence Tomography

OCT is a rapid and noninvasive technique utilized for cross-sectional imaging of the retina. It facilitates the measurement of macular thickness and the detection of macular edema, which is the

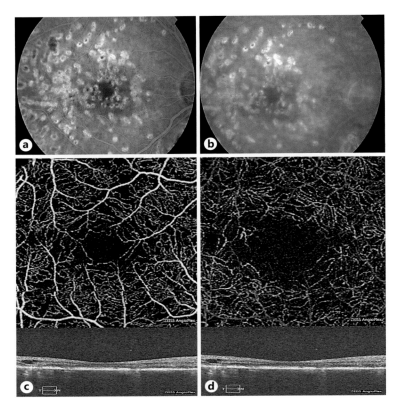

Fig. 3. FA, OCTA and OCT of a patient with proliferative diabetic retinopathy. **a, b** Early- and late-phase FA images show pinpoint hyperfluorescent lesions corresponding to microaneurysms. **c** Three-by-three millimeter OCT angiogram of the superficial capillary plexus and corresponding OCT B-scan, demonstrating enlargement of the FAZ, vascular tortuosity and ischemic areas. **d** Three-by-three millimeter OCT angiogram of the deep capillary plexus and corresponding OCT B-scan, showing remodeling of the FAZ, which looks even more enlarged compared to the superficial capillary plexus.

main pathologic feature of diabetic maculopathy [11, 12]. Characteristics of macular edema in OCT, apart from increased retinal thickness, include intra-retinal spaces of reduced reflectivity, disintegration of the retinal layers, and usually, flattening of the central foveal depression. OCT can also show hard exudates as small hyperreflective deposits with posterior shadowing, serous retinal detachment and vitreoretinal traction [13].

Thus, OCT may assist with the selection of patients with diabetic maculopathy who can benefit from treatment, the identification of which treatment is indicated and precise monitoring of the treatment response. It seems to be the technique of choice for the early detection of diabetic macular abnormalities and the quantification of their reductions after treatment.

Optical Coherence Tomography Angiography
OCTA is a relatively new noninvasive imaging technique used to visualize ocular blood flow in the retinal and choroidal vascular networks. It is a dye-free, rapid, three-dimensional method, unlike traditional FA and indocyanine green angiography.

OCTA is based on algorithms that convert multiple A-scans to OCTA images. OCT angiograms are co-registered with OCT B-scans that are obtained concurrently, allowing for visualization of both retinal flow and structure in tandem. In DR, OCTA is useful for locating and measuring the sizes of different alterations, such as exudates, microaneurysms and microhemorrhages, and it allows for the visualization of foveal microvascular changes that are not detected by clinical examination in diabetic eyes [14].

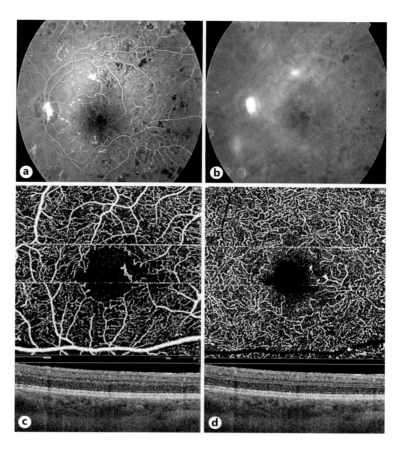

Fig. 4. FA, OCTA and OCT of a patient with nonproliferative diabetic retinopathy. **a, b** Early- and late-phase FA images show microaneurysms and hypofluorescence between the retinal vessels and nonperfused retinal areas, and the capillaries located adjacent to these areas of ischemia are dilated. **c** Three-by-three millimeter OCT angiogram of the superficial capillary plexus and corresponding OCT B-scan, showing enlargement of the FAZ, vascular tortuosity and ischemic areas not seen on FA. **d** Three-by-three millimeter OCT angiogram of the deep capillary plexus and corresponding OCT B-scan, showing remodeling of the FAZ, which looks even more enlarged compared to the superficial capillary plexus, and much more subtle areas of capillary nonperfusion.

Three-by-three and six-by-six millimeter OCTA images are comparable for detecting and evaluating the general characteristics of DR and the size of the affected area, but 3 × 3 mm images provide much more details of different vascular features.

CIRRUS HD-OCT model 5000 (Carl Zeiss Meditec, Inc., United States) and DRI OCT TRITON (Triton, Topcon, Inc., Tokyo, Japan) have been used to obtain OCTA images (figures 1–4). OCTA may provide new information about disease pathophysiology, in addition to being a safe, noninvasive, and viable substitute for dye angiography.

In the literature, comparisons among OCTA, dye angiography and OCT imaging have also been described. Future studies including patients with variable demographics and larger sample sizes for higher-powered determinations of sensitivity and specificity are necessary to evaluate the robustness of this technique in the evaluation of various forms of DR.

Conclusion

OCTA is an emerging technology that allows for the detection of angiographic features of DR and changes in the macular capillary network, even before disease onset. It can show much greater detail compared with FA of microaneurysms, enlarged foveal avascular zones, areas of retinal nonperfusion, reduced capillary density, capillary tortuosity and dilatation, identifying their locations in the superficial and deep capillary plexuses. It cannot show leakage but can better delineate areas of capillary drop-out and detect early retinal neovascularization. OCTA may be useful in the near future for the earlier diagnosis and better management of DR.

References

1 Nentwich MM, Ulbing MW: Diabetic retinopathy – ocular complications of diabetes mellitus. World J Diabetes 2015;6:489–499.

2 Jau JW, Rogers SL, Kawasaki R, et al: Global prevalence and major risk factors of diabetic retinopathy. Diabetes Care 2012;35:556–564.

3 Do DV, Wang X, Vedula SS, et al: Blood pressure control for diabetic retinopathy. Cochrane Database Syst Rev 2015; 1:CD006127.

4 Bandello F, Lattanzio R, Zucchiatti I, et al: Non-proliferative diabetic retinopathy; in Bandello F, Zarbin MA, Lattanzio R, Zucchiatti I (eds): Clinical Strategies in the Management of Diabetic Retinopathy. Berlin Heidelberg, Springer, 2014, pp 19–63.

5 Newman DK: Surgical management of the late complications of proliferative diabetic retinopathy. Eye 2010;24:441–449.

6 Salz DA, Witkin AJ: Imaging in diabetic retinopathy. Middle East Afr J Ophthalmol 2015;22:145–150.

7 Aiello L, Berrocal J, David M, et al: The diabetic retinopathy study. Arch Ophthalmol 1973;90:347–348.

8 Early Treatment Diabetic Retinopathy Study Research Group: Treatment techniques and clinical guidelines for photocoagulation of diabetic macular edema: ETDRS report no. 11. Ophthalmology 1987;94:761–774.

9 Early Treatment Diabetic Retinopathy Study Research Group: Classification of diabetic retinopathy from fluorescein angiograms: ETDRS report no. 2. Ophthalmology 1991;98:807–822.

10 Wessel MM, Aaker GD, Parlitsis G, et al: Ultra-wide-field angiography improves the detection and classification of diabetic retinopathy. Retina 2012;32:785–791.

11 Lattanzio R, Brancato R, Pierro L, et al: Macular thickness measured by optical coherence tomography (OCT) in diabetic patients. Eur J Ophthalmol 2002;12:482–487.

12 Querques G, Lattanzio R, Querques L, et al: Enhanced depth imaging optical coherence tomography in type 2 diabetes. Invest Ophthalmol Vis Sci 2012;53:6017–6024.

13 Sikorski BL, Malukiewicz G, Stafiej J, et al: The diagnostic function of OCT in diabetic maculopathy. Mediators Inflamm 2013;2013:434560.

14 De Carlo TE, Chin AT, Filho MAB, et al: Detection of microvascular changes in eyes of pathients with diabetes but not clinical diabetic retinopathy using optical coherence tomography angiography. Retina 2015;35:2364–2370.

Giuseppe Querques
Department of Ophthalmology, University Vita-Salute
San Raffaele Scientific Institute, Via Olgettina 60
IT–20132 Milan (Italy)
E-Mail querques.giuseppe@hsr.it

Bandello F, Souied EH, Querques G (eds): OCT Angiography in Retinal and Macular Diseases.
Dev Ophthalmol. Basel, Karger, 2016, vol 56, pp 113–121 (DOI: 10.1159/000442802)

New Findings in Diabetic Maculopathy and Proliferative Disease by Swept-Source Optical Coherence Tomography Angiography

Paulo E. Stanga[a–c] · Alessandro Papayannis[a, b] · Emmanouil Tsamis[a–c] · Francesco Stringa[a] · Tim Cole[d] · Yvonne D'Souza[a–c] · Assad Jalil[a, b]

[a]Manchester Vision Regeneration (MVR) Lab at Manchester Royal Eye Hospital & NIHR/Wellcome Trust Manchester CRF, Manchester, [b]Manchester Royal Eye Hospital, Central Manchester University Hospitals NHS Foundation Trust, Manchester, [c]Institute of Human Development, Faculty of Medical and Human Sciences, University of Manchester, Manchester, [d]Topcon (GB) Ltd., Newbury, UK

Abstract

Purpose: To describe the optical coherence tomography (OCT) angiography (OCTA) features of diabetic retinopathy. **Methods:** Retrospective serial case reports were examined of patients who underwent routine clinical examination and OCTA with both DRI OCT Atlantis prototype and Triton Swept-Source OCT of the posterior pole and mid-periphery. When considered necessary, fluorescein fundus angiography (FFA) with OPTOS California wide-field imaging was performed. The findings were compared with the current literature. **Results:** Forty-three consecutive patients (86 eyes) were evaluated. Fourteen of these patients (28 eyes) underwent an additional FFA examination due to advanced retinopathy signs, such as diabetic macular edema, ischemia or neovascularization (NV). OCTA was able to detect the microvascular lesions observed on color fundus images in the whole sample. Thirty-six of the 86 eyes showed foveal avascular zone enlargement on OCTA. Microvascular lesions, diabetic macular edema, and NV of the optic disc observed on FFA were also detected on OCTA in all cases (28/28 eyes). Features of NV elsewhere were detected on FFA in 16/28 eyes. Ten of the 16 eyes had signs of NV within the 100 central degrees, and OCTA was able to detect these signs in 9 of the eyes. **Conclusion:** OCTA is an effective noninvasive imaging technique that can provide additional information regarding the localization and morphology of vascular lesions in all cases of NV of the optic disc and in more than half of cases of NV elsewhere, suggesting that it is a noninferior technique for the study of posterior pole alterations compared with FFA, which remains the gold standard and is fundamental for the study of the retinal periphery.

© 2016 S. Karger AG, Basel

Introduction

Diabetic retinopathy (DR) is the leading cause of blindness in the working population in industrially developed countries [1, 2]. The diagnosis, treatment planning and follow-up of DR are currently based on imaging provided by fluorescein fundus angiography (FFA) and optical coherence tomography (OCT) [3, 4].

FFA is a well-known technique [5, 6] and is currently the gold standard for evaluating the clinical fundus features of DR [7]. It involves the use of fluorescein dye injection to obtain a vascular map of the eye, thereby revealing signs of initial DR, including primary vascular lesions, such as microaneurysms, and vascular abnormalities, such as venous beading and intraretinal microvascular abnormalities. Moreover, it can reveal signs of advanced DR, such as ischemia and neovascularization (NV). Peripheral retinal nonperfusion, which represents intraretinal capillary occlusion or dropout, can be observed as a dark area surrounded by large retinal vessels. New vessels can be identified by remarkable leakage of the dye into the surrounding retinal tissue.

In the macular area, FFA can provide detailed visualization of the breakdown of the inner hematoretinal barrier that leads to diabetic macular edema and enlargement of the foveal avascular zone, which is significantly larger in diabetic eyes compared to healthy eyes [8, 9].

The main advantage of FFA is that it provides pan-retinal imaging of vascular alterations due to DR. This faculty is of great importance in the management of proliferative DR. However, FFA has two important limitations.

First, it is an invasive method that requires intravenous dye injection. Systemic vascular complications, such as severe renal and cardiovascular diseases, are often present in patients with severe DR, while nausea and rarely, anaphylaxis, can occur, even in healthy subjects. Therefore, caution is required when injecting patients for FFA purposes [10, 11].

Another disadvantage of FFA is that it produces bi-dimensional images in which the fluorescence signals of the superficial and deep capillary networks overlap. The inability to visualize the structures of the major capillary networks on a layer-by-layer basis results in a lack of information on the different segmented retinal layers (i.e. segmentation of the retinal layers).

Optical coherence tomography angiography (OCTA) is a quick, standardized, and easily repeatable technique that does not require dye injection, which is an advantage over FFA. However, it does not provide direct information regarding the status of vascular disease or allow for the evaluation of lesions at the extreme retinal periphery.

Newly developed OCTA techniques, such as swept-source OCT with high-speed scanning, can be used to visualize the pathologic vascular changes of DR, with particular focus on microaneurysms, retinal nonperfusion, and NV. Images from wide-field 12 × 9 mm scans or composite images from 6 × 6 mm scans, if appropriately prepared, can represent reproducible images of vascular lesions caused by DR up to the mid-periphery (like FFA) and can provide additional three-dimensional information regarding the localization and morphology of vascular lesions in DR, not only inside of different retinal layers (i.e. retinal segmentation) but also in the vitreous cavity (i.e. vitreous segmentation) (unlike FAA).

The purpose of this chapter is to describe the OCTA features in DR, with introductions of new terms and concepts, to our knowledge, such as peripheral retinal analysis and vitreous segmentation, for descriptive analyses of this complicated pan-retinal disease.

Foveal Avascular Zone Enlargement, Macular Ischemia and Microvascular Alterations

OCTA can allow for the noninvasive visualization of enlargement of the foveal avascular zone (fig. 1) with higher definition compared to conventional FFA, permitting visualization of ischemic alterations in the depth of the retina, with layer-by-layer analysis of the different retinal vascular plexuses [12, 13]. The benefits of such a segmented evaluation can also be applied for local-

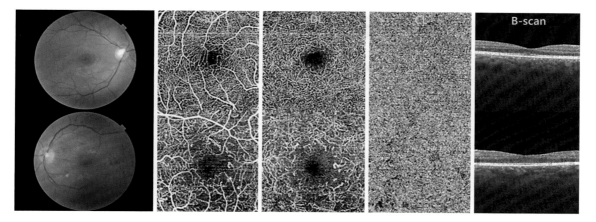

Fig. 1. Fundus color photographs; optical coherence tomography (OCT) angiography (OCTA) images of the outer, inner and choriocapillary vascular plexuses and OCT B-scan images of two 30-year-old male subjects. Top row: healthy eye. Bottom row: nonproliferative diabetic retinopathy (DR) with microvascular alterations and enlargement of the foveal avascular zone.

ization of the origins of microvascular alterations (i.e. microaneurysms) within the superficial and/ or deep neurovascular layers. Some well-demarcated vascular alterations can be better visualized on OCTA than on FFA; inversely, some rare dot-like hyperfluorescent FFA spots cannot be attributed to precise microvascular alterations in OCTA images after analysis with automated segmentation. In such cases, manual segmentation may reveal the origins of these spots, even if, in general, no alterations can be observed in the outer retina [14]. Another explanation for this discrepancy between the two techniques in these rare cases may be extremely slow (i.e. below the sensitivity limit) or fast (i.e. above the saturation limit) blood flow in these specific microvascular alterations during acquisition, resulting in no signal or a saturated decorrelation signal, respectively (fig. 1, 2).

Diabetic Macular Edema and Hard Exudates

Pseudocystic spaces inside of the retina due to diabetic macular edema appear as hypo-reflective, dark areas predominantly located inside of the

deep neurovascular layer of segmentation (fig. 3). This aspect is justified by the absence of blood flow inside of these spaces (excessively low decorrelation signal). Associated microvascular alterations in both the superficial and deep vascular layers and/or retinal ischemia are commonly present.

On the contrary, hard exudates appear as intense hyper-reflective areas in outer retinal segmentation angiograms (fig. 4). This intense hyper-reflective behavior of this substance is defined as a nonvascular decorrelation signal. This signal is generated by structures in which blood does not move, and it might be generated from very small eye motion or by OCT scanning changes produced by these small structures [15].

Evaluation of Peripheral Neovascularization and Ischemia

OCTA, if appropriately used, can provide a scan of the mid-periphery of the retina, highlighting significant vascular alterations, such as the presence of ischemia and NV (fig. 5–7), and can be a helpful guide both before and after surgical or clinical treatments [16].

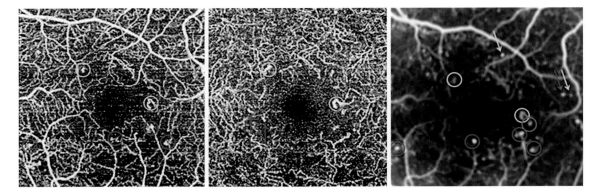

Fig. 2. Detailed analysis of 3 × 3 mm standardized macular OCTA scans of the superficial (left) and deep (center) vascular layers in comparison with a fluorescein fundus angiography (FFA) image (right) of the diabetic eye described in figure 1. The red circles indicate microvascular alterations on FFA, the origins of which are defined in the superficial vascular layer on OCTA. The blue circles highlight lesions originating in the deep vascular layer. The yellow circles show vascular abnormalities derived from both layers matching those on FFA. The arrows point to lesions that are better visualized using one technique over the other (yellow: better visualization with FFA; and green: better with OCTA). The red arrow highlights a hyperfluorescent spot that cannot be matched with any hyper-reflective alteration on OCTA.

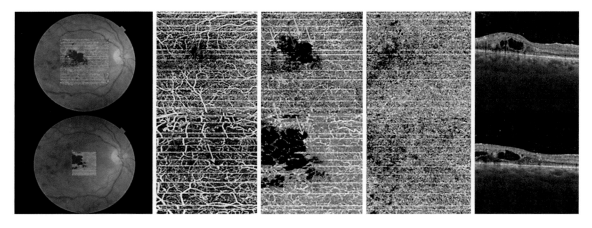

Fig. 3. OCTA angiograms (6 × 6 mm (top row) and 3 × 3 mm (bottom row)) of a 20-year-old female patient with advanced proliferative DR. From left to right: color fundus images with overlying outer vascular network and outer and inner vascular networks, choriocapillary angiograms, and B-scan OCT image. The red arrows show hypo-reflective areas due to presence of diabetic macular edema, the yellow arrows point to the associated microvascular alterations, and the green arrows indicate areas of associated ischemic alterations of both the superficial and inner vascular networks that are also associated with choriocapillary network rarefaction, as indicated by the blue arrows.

Segmentation of the Vitreous

Adequate segmentation of the vitreous is necessary for visualization of new vessels in the superficial retinal layer or in the depth of the vitreous cavity. We illustrate two types of semi-automated segmentation.

DRI OCT-1 Atlantis Swept-Source OCT prototype offers the option to segment the vitreous after flattening of the retina at the inner limiting

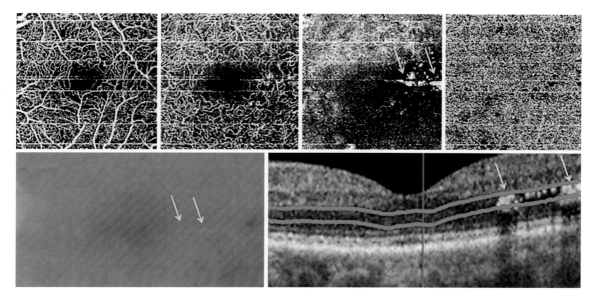

Fig. 4. OCT angiogram of hard exudates (yellow arrows) evident only in the outer neuroepithelial layer as hyper-reflective areas (second images on the top right) after appropriate manual segmentation, as illustrated in OCT B-scan segmentation image (bottom right).

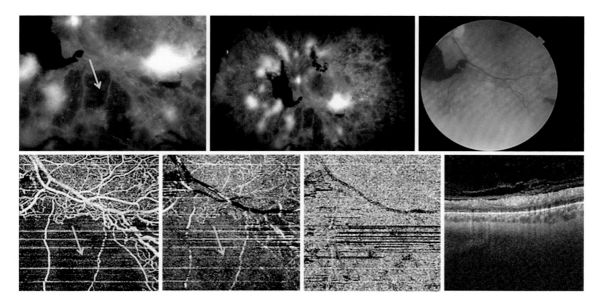

Fig. 5. OCT angiograms of peripheral ischemia (yellow arrows) in a 22-year-old female with severe proliferative DR. From left to the right on the top: FFA and color fundus images. On the bottom: OCT angiograms of the outer vascular network, inner vascular network and choriocapillaris and B-scan OCT image. The red arrows indicate ischemic changes of the choriocapillaris after PASCAL pan-retinal laser treatment.

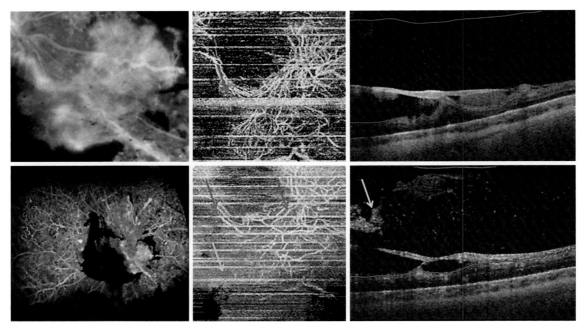

Fig. 6. OCT angiogram showing a fibrovascular membrane growing in the direction of the nasal retina from the optic disc in a 22-year-old woman with severe proliferative DR. OCT angiogram and OCT B-scan at 1 day before intravitreal injection of bevacizumab (top center and right, respectively) and at 3 days after injection (bottom center and right). Early-phase FFA images (left images) showing excessive leakage from the neovascularization (NV) membrane at 1 day before injection. The red arrows point to massive structures of NV in the fibrovascular membrane, which were remarkably reduced in size after anti-vascular endothelial growth factor injection. The yellow arrow shows hemovitreous (due to the mixing of vitreous and epiretinal blood caused by intravitreal injection of bevacizumab) with a subsequent increase in background noise in angiograms obtained after the intravitreal injection of Avastin. The upper green line shows details of manual vitreous cavity segmentation at 1,100 μm inside of the vitreous core, with the lower band settled on the inner limiting membrane (ILM).

membrane layer, followed by analysis of a segment of variable width as needed by the user (yellow bands in fig. 8, 9). This capability allows for segmentation of the superficial retinal layer in association with the outer vitreous cavity or of vitreous segments of various depths, thereby achieving tri-dimensional analysis of the vessels (fig. 8, 9).

DRI OCT Triton Swept-Source OCT offers another type of semi-automated segmentation. The user has to adjust the lower segmentation band in a retinal layer, such as the inner plexiform layer/inner nuclear layer (fig. 10, 11) or inner limiting membrane (fig. 7), and the upper band can be adjusted according to the desired depth of study, generating vitreoretinal or outer vitreous segmentation accordingly.

The major limitation of this modality of segmentation is that with increasing proximity to the periphery, the sensitivity of the software for recognizing the outer retinal layers decreases (macular vitreoretinal segmentation in figure 10 versus peripheral vitreoretinal segmentation in fig. 11). Manual segmentation may be needed to improve the quality of images from the mid-extreme periphery [17].

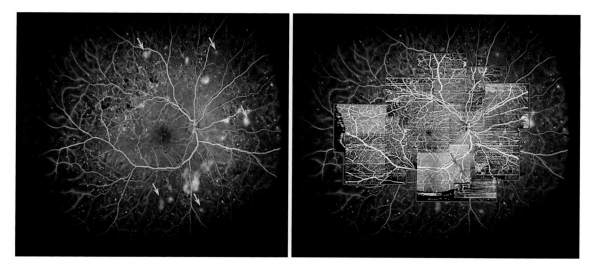

Fig. 7. OCTA composite image of the posterior pole and mid-periphery obtained using DRI OCT Triton Swept-Source with OPTOS California wide-field FFA imaging. The achieved scanned area is defined within the red-colored border on the right image. The red arrows indicate the common sites of NV, and the yellow arrows point to the sites of NV that cannot be detected by OCTA in the extreme periphery.

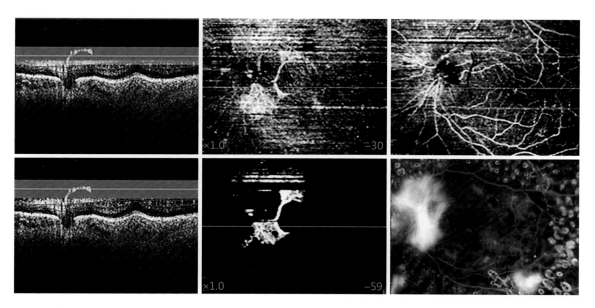

Fig. 8. Left column: OCT B-scan images after ILM flattening, with the segmentation area indicated by the yellow band. Top left: example of vitreoretinal segmentation. Bottom left: example of outer vitreous segmentation. Center column: respective OCTA images. Top right: OCTA image generated after superior retinal segmentation (within the green lines). Bottom right: FFA image.

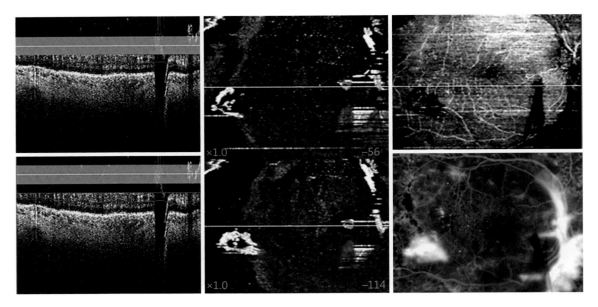

Fig. 9. Left column: OCT B-scan images after ILM flattening, with the segmentation area indicated by the yellow band. Top left: example of outer vitreous segmentation. Bottom left: example of inner vitreous segmentation. Center column: respective OCTA images. Top right: OCTA image generated after superior retinal segmentation (within the green lines). Bottom right: FFA image.

Fig. 10. Example of macular vitreo-retinal segmentation, with the lower segmentation band in the inner plexiform layer/INL and the upper band adjusted at 300 μm inside of the vitreous cavity.

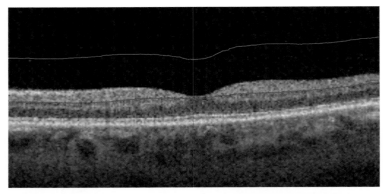

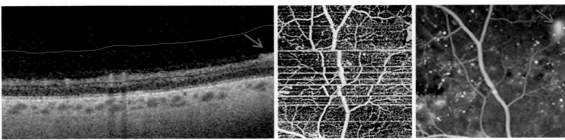

Fig. 11. Example of mid-peripheral vitreoretinal segmentation, with the lower segmentation band in the inner plexiform layer/INL and the upper band adjusted at 300 μm inside of the vitreous cavity. The red arrows indicate neovascularization elsewhere in the OCT B-scan (left), OCTA (center) and FFA (right) images.

Conclusions

OCTA is an effective noninvasive imaging technique that can provide additional three-dimensional information regarding the localization and morphology of vascular lesions in DR due to its unique segmental modality of data acquisition, not only inside of the different retinal layers but also in the vitreous cavity. The currently available OCTA acquisition systems can be used to not only study the macular and optic disc areas but also detect the presence of NV in all cases of NV of the optic disc if properly used, in addition to the majority of cases of NV elsewhere or ischemia affecting the posterior pole and mid-periphery. This capability indicates that OCTA is a noninferior technique for the study of posterior pole alterations compared with FFA, which remains the gold standard and is fundamental for the study of the retinal periphery. Further prospective studies are needed, and new OCTA instruments must be developed that can combine features, such as high-speed scanning, wide-field imaging, eye tracking technology, peripheral acquisition and automated fixation systems, composite imaging and adequate automated segmentation software.

References

1 Klein R, Klein BE, Moss SE, et al: The Wisconsin Epidemiologic Study of Diabetic Retinopathy. III. Prevalence and risk of diabetic retinopathy when age at diagnosis is 30 or more years. Arch Ophthalmol 1984;102:527–532.

2 Antonetti DA, Klein R, Gardner TW: Diabetic Retinopathy. New Engl J Med 2012;366:1227–1239.

3 Buabbud JC, Al-latayfeh MM, Sun JK: Optical coherence tomography imaging for diabetic retinopathy and macular edema. Curr Diab Rep 2010;10:264–269.

4 Norton EW, Gutman F: Diabetic retinopathy studied by fluorescein angiography. Trans Am Ophthalmol Soc 1965; 63:108–128.

5 Flocks M, Miller J, Chao P: Retinal circulation time with the aid of fundus cinephotography. Am J Ophthalmol 1959;48(1, Part 2):3–10.

6 Kikai K: Über die Vitalfärbung des hinteren Bulbusabschnittes. Arch Augenheilkd 1930;103:541–553.

7 Gass JM: A fluorescein angiographic study of macular dysfunction secondary to retinal vascular disease. IV. Diabetic retinal angiopathy. Arch Ophthalmol 1968;80:583–591.

8 Bresnick GH, Condit R, Syrjala S, et al: Abnormalities of the foveal avascular zone in diabetic retinopathy. Arch Ophthalmol 1984;102:1286–1293.

9 Conrath J, Giorgi R, Raccah D, et al: Foveal avascular zone in diabetic retinopathy: quantitative vs qualitative assessment. Eye (Lond) 2005;19:322–326.

10 Cheung N, Wang JJ, Klein R, et al: Diabetic retinopathy and the risk of coronary heart disease: the Atherosclerosis Risk in Communities Study. Diabetes Care 2007;30:1742–1746.

11 Kawasaki R, Cheung N, Islam FM, et al: Is diabetic retinopathy related to subclinical cardiovascular disease? Ophthalmology 2011;118:860–865.

12 Freiberg FJ, Pfau M, Wons J, et al: Optical coherence tomography angiography of the foveal avascular zone in diabetic retinopathy. Graefes Arch Clin Exp Ophthalmol 2015, Epub ahead of print.

13 Di G, Weihong Y, Xiao Z, et al: A morphological study of the foveal avascular zone in patients with diabetes mellitus using optical coherence tomography angiography. Graefes Arch Clin Exp Ophthalmol 2015, Epub ahead of print.

14 Ishibazawa A, Nagaoka T, Takahashi A, et al: Optical coherence tomography angiography in diabetic retinopathy: a prospective pilot study. Am J Ophthalmol 2015;160:35–44.e1.

15 Lumbroso BH, Huang D, Chen CJ, et al: Clinical OCT Angriography Atlas. New Delhi, India, Jaypee Brothers Medical Publishers, 2015.

16 Papayannis A, Tsamis E, Stringa F, Chwiejczak K, Cole T, D'Souza Y, Jalil A, Stanga PE: Ultra-wide field sweptsource optical coherence tomography angiography (UWF SS OCT-A) in diabetic retinopathy. Seattle, 2016 ARVO Annual Meeting, Research: A Vision of Hope, May 1–5, 2016.

17 Stanga PE, Jalil A, Tsamis E, Stringa F, Papayannis A: Vitreous segmentation of ocular coherence tomography angiography of the posterior pole and mid-periphery in diabetic retinopathy. Birmingham, RCOphth Annual Congress 2016, May 24–26, 2016.

Paulo E. Stanga
Manchester Vision Regeneration (MVR) Lab
Research Office, Purple Zone, MRI
Central Manchester University Hospitals NHS, Foundation Trust
Oxford Road, Manchester M13 9WL (UK)
E-Mail Paulo.Stanga@cmft.nhs.uk

Bandello F, Souied EH, Querques G (eds): OCT Angiography in Retinal and Macular Diseases.
Dev Ophthalmol. Basel, Karger, 2016, vol 56, pp 122–131 (DOI: 10.1159/000442803)

Optical Coherence Tomography Angiography of Retinal Artery Occlusion

Caroline R. Baumal

Tufts University School of Medicine, New England Eye Center, Boston, Mass., USA

Abstract

The optical coherence tomography angiography (OCTA) microvascular features of branch and central retinal artery occlusion are described and correlated with fluorescein angiographic and clinical findings. There may be differences in the distribution of reduced vascular perfusion/ flow between the superficial and deep retinal capillary plexuses in retinal artery occlusive disease. The extent of macular ischemia and the status of flow in the radial peripapillary capillaries can be evaluated with OCTA. Overall, OCTA can be used to monitor changes in vascular flow during the clinical course of retinal artery occlusion.

© 2016 S. Karger AG, Basel

Accurate and timely diagnosis of nonarteritic retinal artery occlusion (RAO) is critical as it may be the initial presenting sign in individuals at risk of morbidity from systemic embolic events. Individuals with RAO typically present with unilateral, painless sudden loss of vision or scotoma due interruption of the blood supply to the retina. The incidence of central retinal artery occlusion (CRAO) has been estimated to be 1 in 100,000 [1]. Branch retinal artery occlusion (BRAO) usually results from embolic obstruction of a division of the retinal artery, while CRAO results from occlusion of the retinal artery either before it branches at or proximal to the optic disc. There are 2 main arterial systems that supply blood to the retina and choroid. The ophthalmic artery is the first branch of the internal carotid artery and enters the orbit underneath the optic nerve through the optic canal. The central retinal artery (CRA) is the first intraorbital branch of the ophthalmic artery, and it passes into the optic nerve at 8–15 mm behind the globe to supply blood to the inner retina. The CRA measures 160 microns in diameter and leads to four capillary networks within the eye [2]. The radial peripapillary capillaries (RPCs) make up the most superficial capillary layer located in the inner part of the nerve fiber layer, and they run along the paths of the major superotemporal and inferotemporal vessels at 4–5 mm from the optic disk. The RPCs anastomose with each other and with the deeper capillaries. The superficial retinal capillary plexus is located in the nerve fiber layer near the disc (continuous with the RPC system) but is present more predominantly within the ganglion cell layer in the central macular region. The deep retinal capillary plexus is composed of intermediate and deep plexuses located at the inner and outer planes of the inner nuclear layer, respectively [2]. These capillary layers are interconnected by perpendicularly oriented vessels. Layers of the retinal vasculature may be differentially affected by ischemic retinal vascular disease.

The terminal branches of the CRA provide the only blood supply to the inner retina. Of note, the foveola receives its blood supply from the choroidal circulation and is not supplied by the CRA or its branches. The choroid receives its blood supply from the short posterior ciliary arteries that branch distally from the ophthalmic artery. An important anatomical variation noted in 15–20% of the population is a cilioretinal artery that branches from the short posterior ciliary arteries (choroidal circulation). When present, the cilioretinal artery may provide additional blood supply to the retina between the macula and optic nerve (to the papillomacular bundle region), including the nerve fibers from the foveal photoreceptors. If this artery is present, a small area of central vision may be preserved in eyes with CRAO. However, it is also possible for the cilioretinal artery to occlude in isolation (or secondary to central retinal vein occlusion), causing central visual loss with a perfused macula region.

Acute obstruction of the retinal artery with secondary collapse of capillary flow leads to axoplasmic stasis, intracellular edema and ischemic necrosis of the inner retinal layers. This causes the nerve fiber layer and inner retina to become opacified, glassy and whitened in appearance. This opacification is the densest in the posterior pole as a result of increased thickness of the nerve fiber layer and ganglion cells in this area. The fo-

veola assumes a 'cherry-red spot' appearance because the foveolar region is nourished by the choroidal circulation, and thus, the retinal pigment epithelium and choroid remain intact underneath the fovea while the surrounding retina opacifies (fig. 1a). If the CRA becomes occluded, complete loss of vision occurs even though the central foveolar circulation is not affected because the emanating nerve fiber layer is ischemic. Opacification takes as little as 15 min to several hours before becoming apparent. Pigmentary changes are typically absent since the retinal pigment epithelium remains unaffected. A boxcar appearance of the blood column can be seen in both arteries and veins. Hayreh [3] has demonstrated irreversible cell injury after 90 min of CRAO in primates. The clinical appearance of retinal whitening resolves in 4–6 weeks. The obstructed retinal artery may eventually recanalize and reperfuse, with resolution of the inner retinal edema. However, the inner retinal damage is permanent, leading to atrophy, retinal vascular attenuation and optic nerve pallor. During the late stage of RAO, marked inner retinal thinning occurs due to ischemia. Vision and/or field loss often do not recover after RAO because the retinal damage becomes established quickly, and there is no effective way to reverse the obstruction. Methods to lower the intraocular pressure and/or dislodge the embolus include anterior chamber paracentesis, administration of intraocular pressure-lowering drops, ocular massage and intra-arterial tissue plasminogen activator with a conservative treatment window of 24 hours after RAO.

It is usually not difficult to diagnose RAO clinically during the acute phase when retinal opacification is obvious. However, this sign may not be obvious very early in the course of RAO, in eyes with partial RAO or at 4–6 weeks after RAO has occurred. Ancillary testing with intravenous fluorescein angiography (FA) and spectral-domain optical coherence tomography (SD-OCT) is useful to evaluate the extent of retinal nonperfusion, to search for other vascular abnormalities and to

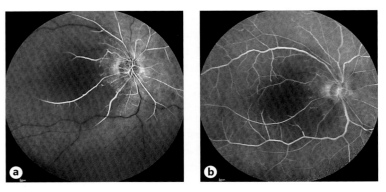

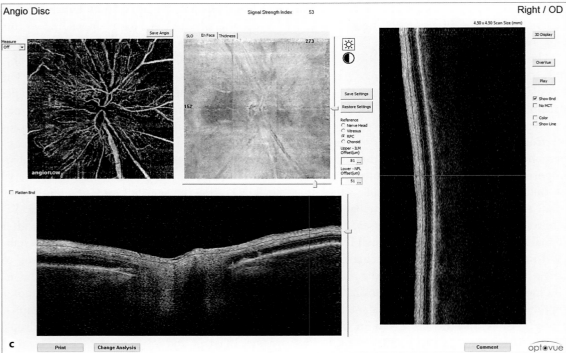

Fig. 1. a, **b** Stages of chronic central retinal artery occlusion (CRAO) in the right eye. Visual acuity measured hand motions. Fluorescein angiogram of the right eye at 60 seconds (1a) and 5 minutes (1b) during the acute phase of CRAO. **c** Relative sparing of the radial peripapillary capillaries in acute CRAO, as demonstrated by optical coherence tomography (OCT) angiography (OCTA) centered over the optic nerve. **d** OCTA in acute CRAO revealed severely impaired flow in both the superficial and deep retinal capillary plexuses and inner retinal thickening on OCT B-scan. **e** At 8 weeks following acute CRAO, OCTA demonstrated increased flow visible on the superficial and deep retinal capillary scans.

(For figure 1d, e see next page.)

Baumal

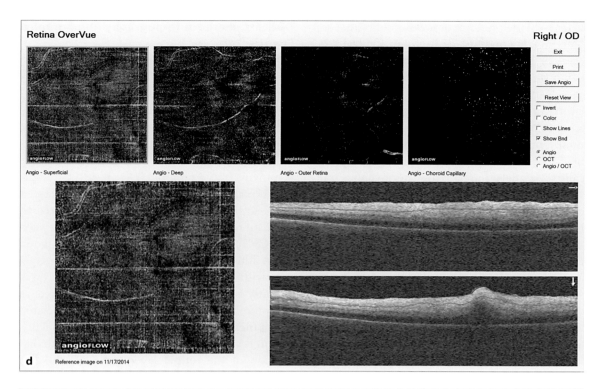

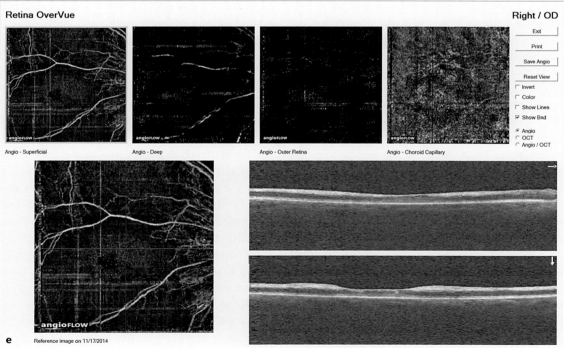

determine the presence or location of retinal emboli. Imaging may also be useful in atypical RAO cases or if acute signs are not apparent. FA depends on the dynamic properties of blood flow to show early and late changes in the retinal vasculature. In the acute setting, FA delineates the extent of involvement of the retina, seen as capillary nonperfusion and absent or delayed filling of the blood vessels distal to the obstruction. It specifically shows delays in both the arteriovenous transit time and retinal arterial filling with normal choroidal filling. Ophthalmic artery or carotid artery obstruction should be considered if there is delayed choriocapillaris filling. After resolution and recanalization of acute CRAO, FA may show arterial narrowing with normal fluorescein transit. It mainly provides information about large vessel flow but does not allow for assessment of the morphology of the deep capillary network. In addition, assessment of the deeper retinal capillaries with FA may be limited by light scattering from the opacified inner retinal layers. SD-OCT can be utilized to determine the specific retinal level of edema or subsequent atrophy during the chronic phase, when FA may no longer show any perfusion deficit [4–6].

Optical coherence tomography angiography (OCTA) may have advantages over other imaging techniques for eyes with nonarteritic RAO. OCTA enables three-dimensional and *en face* visualization of flow in the retinal and choroidal vasculature. Thus, it can reveal deficiencies involving acute flow interruption in RAO. In addition, it provides *en face* segmented imaging of the deep vascular plexus, which is poorly imaged with FA, and reveals finer details of the superficial vascular plexus [7]. Precise localization of retinal capillary ischemia with OCTA in RAO may help to determine subsequent visual prognosis. OCTA is dye-free, which may be beneficial for patients with concomitant medical problems who may not be able to tolerate dye-based angiography.

Optical Coherence Tomography Angiography Features

The utility of *en face* OCTA to characterize vascular flow changes related to RAO in the superficial and deep retinal capillary systems and in the RPCs has been characterized using prototype AngioVue SD-OCTA software within the commercially available RTVue XR Avanti device (Optovue Inc., Fremont, CA) [8, 9]. Three-dimensional OCT angiograms and co-registered cross-sectional OCT B-scans can be utilized to evaluate retinal flow and structure, respectively. The OCTA features in RAO have been compared to FA and SD-OCT B-scan findings. A series of 7 eyes with acute or chronic CRAO or BRAO was recently reported. Acute RAO was defined as symptoms lasting for less than 14 days associated with inner retinal whitening, delayed arterial filling on FA and inner retinal thickening, with disruption of the retinal layers on OCT B-scan. Chronic RAO was characterized by a known prior history of acute RAO, with residual narrowed retinal vessels and atrophy of the inner retinal layers on SD-OCT.

OCTA images in RAO revealed variable amounts of decreased vascular perfusion in both the superficial and deep retinal capillary plexuses corresponding to both the areas of delayed perfusion on FA and the inner retinal changes on OCT B-scan (fig. 1–3). In eyes with acute CRAO, OCTA centered at the macula may demonstrate equal areas of decreased vascular perfusion in both the superficial and deep capillary plexuses (fig. 1). In one eye with CRAO and cilioretinal sparing, OCTA revealed a wider area of decreased vascular perfusion in the superficial capillary plexus compared to the deep capillary plexus [8]. Caution should be taken when evaluating deep retinal capillary plexus flow in eyes with acute CRAO as there may be an element of signal attenuation secondary to inner retinal layer optical reflectivity-producing artifacts masking as hypoperfusion. Assessment of co-registered OCT B-

Fig. 2. Features of embolic branch retinal artery occlusion (BRAO) on OCTA compared to fluorescein angiography (FA) in the right eye. Visual acuity was 20/25–2, with a superior visual field defect. Fundoscopic examination showed BRAO with multiple retinal emboli along the inferior arcade, retinal opacification, retinal artery constriction peripheral to the emboli and a cotton wool spot. **a** Fundus photograph of acute BRAO with multiple emboli (arrow), a cotton wool spot (arrowhead) and an opacified ischemic retina. **b** FA (Heidelberg Spectralis, Germany) at 60 s (**A**) demonstrates a severe filling defect in the inferotemporal occluded branch retinal artery. There is early blockage at a retinal artery bifurcation with absent flow distal to the blockage (arrow), retinal capillary nonperfusion and a cotton wool spot (arrowhead). Late-phase FA performed at 6 min (**B**) revealed scanty foci of fluorescein dye in the retinal artery distal to the occlusion and staining of the associated dilated retinal vein. **c** Wide-field image of the right eye created from multiple 3 × 3 mm OCT angiograms using a montage technique. The OCT angiograms are segmented between Bruch's membrane and the inner limiting membrane. The cotton wool spot (arrow) and the site of arterial occlusion (arrowhead) are marked. OCT B-scans at different sites (**B**, **C**) are shown by the dashed lines on the montage. **d** OCT angiograms of the superficial (**A**) and deep (**C**) retinal capillary plexuses. The arrows demarcate the borders of capillary loss and ischemia, which appear larger in the superficial plexus (**A**) than in the deep plexus (**C**). OCT B-scans show the segmentation lines used to create the en face OCTA images of the superficial plexus (**B**) and deep plexus (**D**).

(For figure 2d see next page.)

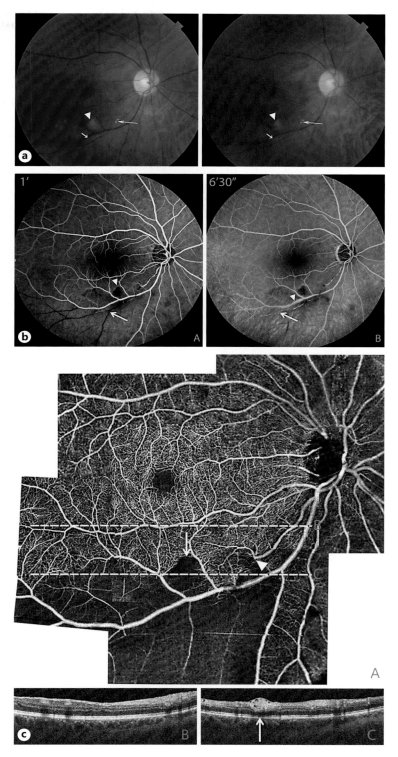

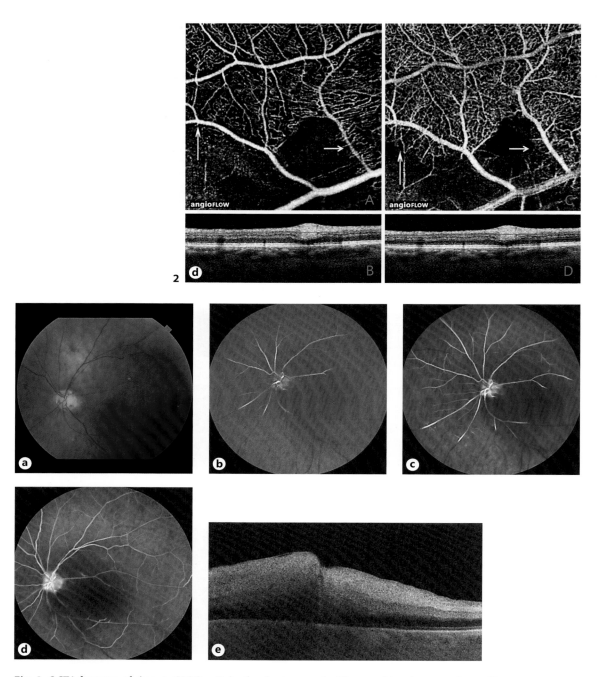

Fig. 3. OCTA features of chronic CRAO. **a** Color fundus image of a 60-year-old male presenting with acute nonarteritic CRAO. **b–d** FA images obtained at the early (3b), middle (3c) and late (3d) phases reveal severely impaired flow. **e** OCT B-scan in acute CRAO reveals severe thickening of the inner retina and loss of retinal architecture due to edema. **f** Automated AngioVue OCTA performed at 3 months after initial presentation with CRAO reveals decreased perfusion in both retinal capillary plexuses. The area of decreased perfusion appears larger in the deep capillary plexus. The OCT B-scan reveals inner retinal atrophy and loss of foveal contour. *(For figure 3f see next page.)*

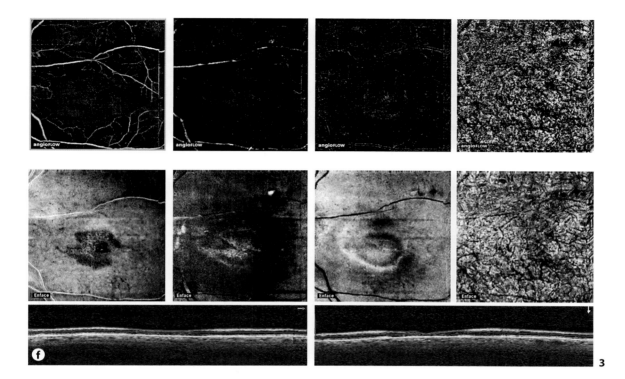

scans may assist in the evaluation of segmentation errors in this scenario.

In 4 eyes with BRAO, 75% of the eyes had a larger area of decreased vascular perfusion in the superficial capillary plexus compared to the deep capillary plexus, while one eye showed a wider area of decreased vascular perfusion in the deep plexus. Figure 2a–d shows OCTA and FA images of acute embolic BRAO. Figure 2c is a montage of multiple 3 × 3 mm OCT angiograms with segmentation between Bruch's membrane and the inner limiting membrane revealing severely decreased flow distal to the obstruction along the inferior arcade and a well-demarcated border of capillary nonperfusion. The retinal capillary nonperfusion is more easily discernable on OCTA than on FA (fig. 2b, c) due to the absence of fluorescein-induced choroidal flush on OCTA. An OCT B-scan peripheral to the occlusion shows inner retinal disorganization,

edema and a cotton wool spot in the nerve fiber layer (fig. 2c, segmentation line C). The segmented OCTA image appears to show a larger area of capillary loss in the superficial retinal capillary plexus compared to the deep plexus, and the border of nonperfusion is well demarcated in the segmented OCTA images (fig. 2d) [9].

During the chronic phase of RAO, flow appears to be re-established in some retinal arterioles on OCTA (fig. 3d). Bonini et al. [8] have hypothesized that reorganization of vascular interconnections in chronic RAO may contribute to partial restoration of deep capillary plexus perfusion in regions where the superficial capillary plexus remains abnormal. OCTA may not always enable differentiation between the superficial and deep retinal plexuses due to extreme inner retinal thinning secondary to the chronic phase after RAO.

OCTA images centered on the optic disc have been used to evaluate the RPC network in eyes with RAO with variable findings (fig. 1c). In CRAO, either preservation or diffuse attenuation of the RPC system has been observed. Eyes with BRAO have been demonstrated focal attenuation of the RPCs distributed in the affected arterial occlusion.

Overall, OCTA in RAO reveals varying severities of vascular nonperfusion in the superficial versus the deep retinal capillary plexus. This finding is in agreement with the results of SD-OCT B-scan studies demonstrating a spectrum of capillary ischemia in retinal artery occlusive disease, ranging from isolated to continuous superficial and/or deep capillary ischemia [5]. It is not clear what factors affect the variations in the location and severity of nonperfusion/ischemia in RAO. One hypothesis is that inner retinal edema during the early stages of RAO causes compression of the ganglion cell and nerve fiber layers, potentially leading to more severe nonperfusion of the superficial capillary plexus. Future studies may elucidate the potential factors affecting the level of retinal ischemia in RAO.

Limitations of Optical Coherence Tomography Angiography in Retinal Artery Occlusion

The use of OCTA to evaluate microvasculature changes in individuals with advanced age, a long axial length, poor vision and retinal vascular disease may have some technical limitations. As OCTA technology is relatively new in the clinical setting, there is currently no large dataset of reproducible findings available comparing normal age-matched subjects to those with ocular disease. Accurate evaluation of the level of retinal capillary ischemia may be limited by patient movement or fixation loss during acquisition, causing reduced image quality. In addition, the structural and optical reflectivity changes resulting from edema and/or atrophy in RAO may affect the accuracy of *en face* segmentation. In a series of RAO eyes studied with OCTA, multiple patients were excluded due to poor image quality resulting from fixation issues [8]. Segmentation failure due to severe retinal atrophy and/or distorted retinal architecture in eyes with chronic RAO may limit assessment of the specific retinal capillary plexuses. In eyes with retinal thinning or high optical intensities of the inner retinal layers, which prohibits *en face* segmentation, assessment of the summed vascular image of the entire inner retina may still provide useful information that parallels FA findings. At present, increasing the size of the area scanned reduces the OCTA flow details. The retinal area affected in RAO can be large and may extend beyond the small OCTA scanning areas. An OCTA montage of 3×3 mm scans can be created manually, as shown in figure 2c, to provide a wider field of view while maintaining microvascular detail. The ability to scan larger areas of the retina with high resolution or to montage multiple scans may become an automatic feature in future OCTA technology. Future advances in OCTA imaging permitting an increased scanning area, a reduction in motion artifacts and a decreased image acquisition time may improve the accuracy of microvasculature imaging in retinal vascular disease and RAO.

Conclusion

OCTA is a useful diagnostic tool used to demonstrate the features necessary to diagnose RAO. Compared to FA, OCTA is fast, noninvasive, and can provide improved visualization of microvascular details. The features of disrupted flow in RAO are apparent with both dynamic FA and static OCTA imaging. Due to the nature of RAO, a static representation is sufficient to make the diagnosis. OCTA can be used to accurately image retinal capillary plexuses at different levels in RAO and may be sufficiently sensitive to demonstrate the extent of ischemia and to monitor vascular flow changes during the disease course. In some eyes with BRAO, OCTA reveals increased disruption of the superficial vascular plexus. The ability of OCTA to visualize fine microvascular changes may allow for the early detection of neovascularization or anastomoses that may arise as a consequence of vascular occlusion.

References

1 Leavitt JA, Larson TA, Hodge DO, et al: The incidence of central retinal artery occlusion in Olmsted County, Minnesota. AJO 2011;152:820–823.
2 Zhang HR: Scanning electron-microscopic study of corrosion casts on retinal and choroidal angioarchitecture in man and animals. Prog Retin Eye Res 1994; 13:243–270.
3 Hayreh SS: Acute retinal arterial occlusive disorders. Prog Retin Eye Res 2011; 30:359–394.
4 Ahn SJ, Woo SJ, Park KH, et al: Retinal and choroidal changes and visual outcome in central retinal artery occlusion: an optical coherence tomography study. Am J Ophthalmol 2015;159:667–676.
5 Yu S, Pang CE, Gong Y, et al: The spectrum of superficial and deep capillary ischemia in retinal artery occlusion. Am J Ophthalmol 2015;159:53–63.e1–e2.
6 Chen H, Chen X, Qiu Z, et al: Quantitative analysis of retinal layers' optical intensities on 3D optical coherence tomography for central retinal artery occlusion. Sci Rep 2015;5:9269.
7 Spaide RF, Klancnik JM Jr, Cooney MJ: Retinal vascular layers imaged by fluorescein angiography and optical coherence tomography angiography. JAMA Ophthalmol 2015;133:45–50.
8 Bonini Filho MA, Adhi M, deCarlo TE, et al: Optical coherence tomography angiography in retinal artery occlusion. Retina 2015;35:2339–2346.
9 de Castro-Abeger AH, de Carlo TE, Duker JS, et al: Optical coherence tomography angiography compared to fluorescein angiography in branch retinal artery occlusion. Ophthalmic Surg Lasers Imaging Retina 2015;46:1052–1054.

Caroline R. Baumal, MD
Tufts University School of Medicine
New England Eye Center
800 Washington Street, Box 450, Boston, MA 02111 (USA)
E-Mail cbaumal@gmail.com

Bandello F, Souied EH, Querques G (eds): OCT Angiography in Retinal and Macular Diseases.
Dev Ophthalmol. Basel, Karger, 2016, vol 56, pp 132–138 (DOI: 10.1159/000442805)

Optical Coherence Tomography Angiography of Retinal Vein Occlusion

Eduardo A. Novais[a, b] · Nadia K. Waheed[b]

[a]Department of Ophthalmology, Federal University of São Paulo, School of Medicine, São Paulo, Brazil;
[b]New England Eye Center at Tufts University School of Medicine, Boston, Mass., USA

Abstract

Retinal vein occlusion is the second most common cause of retinal vascular disease after diabetic retinopathy and is a frequent cause of significant vision loss and associated morbidity. Currently, fluorescein angiography is the gold standard for imaging of the retinal and choroidal vasculature. However, this imaging modality is invasive, involving the use of an intravenous contrast agent that can cause systemic side effects and rarely, anaphylaxis. Optical coherence tomography angiography is a noninvasive, depth-resolved imaging modality that allows for the appreciation of spatial relationships of fundus vessels and enables detailed *en face* visualization of the superficial and deep retinal vasculature separately without the risk of adverse affects associated with the intravenous administration of fluorescein dye. When viewed alongside corresponding structural B-scans, optical coherence tomography angiography demonstrates almost all of the clinical and fluorescein angiographic findings that are characteristic of acute and chronic retinal vein occlusion, such as a decrease in capillary perfusion, macular edema, vascular dilation, foveal avascular zone enlargement, and venous-venous collateral formation.

© 2016 S. Karger AG, Basel

Retinal vein occlusion (RVO) is the second most common cause of retinal vascular disease after diabetic retinopathy and is a frequent cause of significant vision loss and associated morbidity [1–3]. Currently, fluorescein angiography (FA) is the gold standard for imaging of the retinal and choroidal vasculature. It can be used to identify and monitor the development of potentially visually debilitating sequelae of RVO, such as neovascularization and macular edema [4]. However, this imaging modality is invasive and involves the use of intravenous contrast, which can result in systemic side effects and occasionally, in anaphylaxis [5–7].

The retinal capillary network upstream of the retinal veins is arranged in morphologically distinct layers. The superficial retinal capillary plexus is located predominantly within the ganglion cell layer, and the deep retinal capillary plexus is located at the outer boundary of the inner nuclear layer, with a smaller intermediate retinal capillary plexus located at the inner margin of the inner nuclear layer. The vascular layers of the retina are connected by perpendicularly positioned vessels [8]. Evidence suggests that the superficial and deep retinal capillary plexuses may be disproportionately affected in retinal vascular disease [9].

Unlike FA, optical coherence tomography (OCT) angiography (OCTA) is a noninvasive, depth-resolved imaging modality that allows for appreciation of the spatial relationships of fundus vessels and enables detailed *en face* visualization of the superficial and deep retinal vasculature separately without the risk of adverse affects associated with the intravenous administration of fluorescein dye [10, 11]. OCT angiograms can be viewed alongside corresponding structural B-scans to visualize increased central retinal thickness and intraretinal cysts, and these structural findings can be correlated with microvascular details.

The OCTA *en face* acquisition areas currently range from 3 × 3 to 8 × 8 mm for commercially available devices; however, the resolution is decreased in larger scans because the same or a comparable number of B-scans is used across a larger area. Three-by-three millimeter OCT angiograms allow for the visualization of greater microvascular detail than FA or indocyanine green angiography images [12, 13]. In some cases, intensity-based OCTA allows for the visualization of a greater number of capillaries in the pericentral macula than FA [14]. Furthermore, with OCTA, different retinal layers can be resolved, and nonperfusion areas can be easily identified.

Fluorescein Angiography for Retinal Vein Occlusion

On FA, RVO is characterized by delayed venous filling in the region of the obstructed vein, capillary nonperfusion, which may be obscured by retinal hemorrhage, vessel permeability, macular edema, and other microvascular abnormalities, such as microaneurysms, vessel tortuosity and the formation of collateral vessels. FA is used to assess macular edema, the extent of ischemia and the presence of neovascularization, which are findings that can aid clinicians in determining the appropriate treatment. The quality of the image generated by FA depends on the timing of imaging following injection of intravenous sodium fluorescein dye. Importantly, this test cannot be repeated multiple times during a single patient visit and is seldom repeated during follow-up visits due to its invasive nature. Routine follow-up of central retinal vein occlusion (CRVO) generally involves the acquisition of structural OCT scans to determine the presence of edema and to allow for the follow-up of edema with treatment.

There is growing interest in selective visualization of the retinal microvasculature at different capillary levels in retinal vascular disease, as recent studies have identified diseases featuring isolated deep capillary ischemia [15]. The depth and area of decreased vascular perfusion, in addition to the presence or absence of macular edema, may affect the visual prognosis of these eyes. Since FA does not permit individual visualization of the different retinal capillary plexuses, it may fail to recognize deep capillary ischemia [16, 17]. Although retinal vasculature changes in RVO have been described in the literature using conventional imaging techniques such as FA, precise evaluation of the vasculature at different capillary levels is not feasible using FA due to the scattering of fluorescent light, which obscures the view, particularly that of the deep retinal capillary plexus [18].

Optical Coherence Tomography Angiography for Central Retinal Vein Occlusion

OCT B-scans are widely used to qualitatively and quantitatively evaluate retinal thickness to monitor the effectiveness of various treatment modalities and to confirm the resolution of macular edema in CRVO. However, it is not able to identify vascular changes.

With its high-density scanning, OCTA can be used to identify changes in the superficial and deep retinal vascular plexuses that would normally be obscured in FA due to leakage. Avascular areas on FA correspond to dark areas of no flow on OCTA, with decreased flow being more prom-

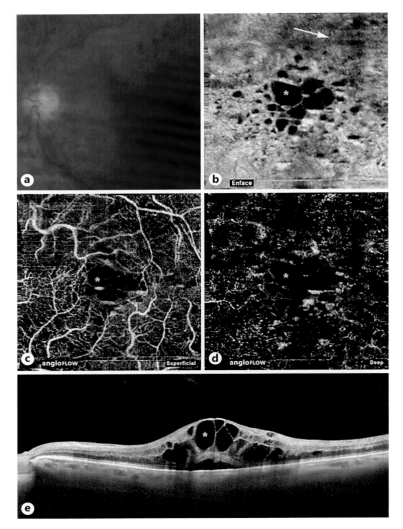

Fig. 1. Seventy-eight-year old Caucasian male with acute central retinal vein occlusion. **a** Color fundus photograph demonstrates intraretinal hemorrhages, dilated tortuous retinal veins, macular edema, and mild optic disc edema. **b** *En face* optical coherence tomography (OCT) shows an area of hyporeflectivity (white arrow) that could contribute to artifactual changes on OCT angiogram. The yellow arrow demonstrates normal reflectivity. The central hyporeflective oblong areas correspond to intraretinal cysts (yellow asterisk). **c** OCT angiogram of the superficial plexus demonstrates attenuation of the OCT angiography signal from the superficial layer, with a nonspecific vascular distribution. **d** OCT angiogram of the deep plexus vasculature demonstrates more extensive loss of capillary blood flow. **e** OCT B-scan. Hyporeflective areas of intraretinal fluid through the fovea do not demonstrate OCT angiography signals (yellow asterisk).

inent in the deep vascular plexus [13]. In the superficial plexus, vessels that are close to the foveal avascular zone (FAZ) are more tortuous and narrowed. Vascular looping, collaterals, telangiectatic vessels, vessel thickening, and focally dilated microaneurysms at the borders of ischemic areas are also easily identified using this technology and are often present in both superficial and deep vascular plexuses. Cystoid macular edema appears as round dark areas with smooth borders on OCTA (fig. 1). It has been reported that edema is related to decreased perfusion of the superficial and deep plexuses on OCTA [13]. However, decreased blood flow on OCTA can be observed even without intraretinal edema in patients with CRVO.

OCTA of chronic CRVO consistently demonstrates diffuse capillary nonperfusion, an enlarged FAZ (fig. 2), telangiectatic vessels, and optociliary shunts (fig. 3). Most importantly, the OCTA image is cross-registered with structural OCT scans that can provide retinal thickness information and

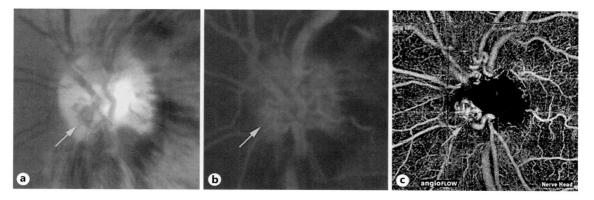

Fig. 2. Fifty-nine-year old African female with central retinal vein occlusion. **a** Color fundus photograph of the optic nerve demonstrates intraretinal hemorrhages and optociliary shunts (yellow arrow). **b** Mid-late-phase fluorescein angiography demonstrates hypofluorescence around the optic nerve secondary to intraretinal hemorrhage blockage and optociliary shunts (yellow arrow). **c** OCT angiogram of the optic nerve demonstrates well-delineated optociliary shunts (yellow arrow).

Fig. 3. Sixty-seven-year old Caucasian male with chronic central retinal vein occlusion. **a** OCT angiogram of the superficial plexus demonstrates attenuation of perifoveal blood flow and foveal avascular zone enlargement (yellow dotted line). **b** OCT angiogram of the deep plexus vasculature demonstrates more extensive loss of capillary blood flow and greater foveal avascular zone enlargement compared to the superficial plexus (red dotted line). **c** Horizontal OCT B-scan centered on the fovea demonstrates an atrophic retina and abnormal retinal layers.

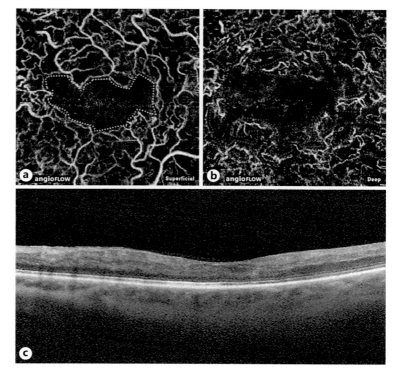

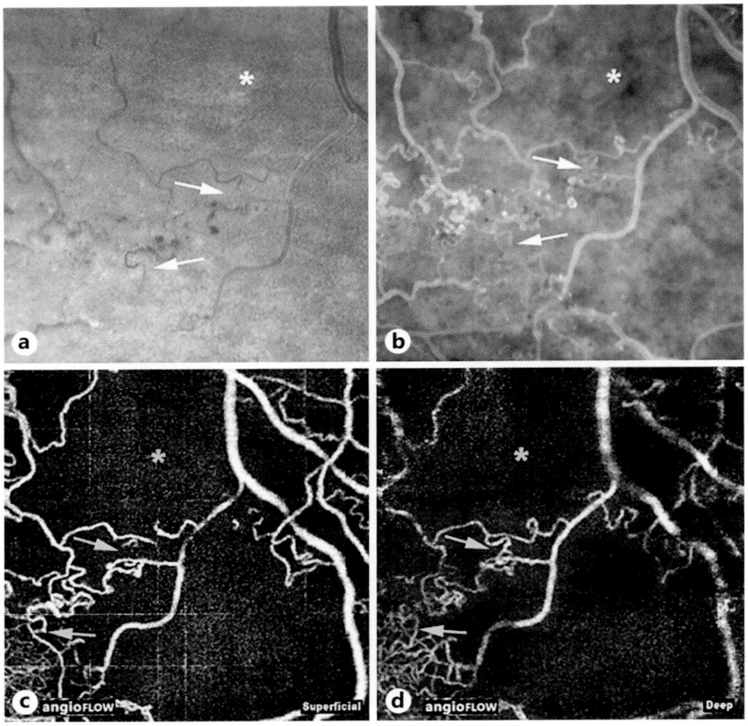

Fig. 4. Sixty-year-old Caucasian male with branch retinal vein occlusion. **a** Color fundus photograph demonstrates an avascular retina (white asterisk) and collateral vessels (white arrows). **b** Mid-late-phase fluorescein angiography demonstrates hypofluorescence from an ischemic retina (white asterisk) and collateral vessels (white arrows). **c, d** OCT angiogram of the superficial and deep plexuses demonstrating an avascular retina (yellow asterisk) and venous-venous anastomosis between the superficial and deep plexuses (yellow arrows).

demonstrate the structural changes such as cystic edema that are essential for making management decisions for patients with CRVO.

Optical Coherence Tomography Angiography for Branch Retinal Vein Occlusion

Vascular changes in branch retinal vein occlusion (BRVO) include changes in vessel caliber and tortuous, narrowed, focally dilated vascular changes. Truncated vessels are shown on OCTA with abrupt interruptions, with terminal dilations at the site of occlusion. By depth-resolved analysis, OCTA allows for visualization of arteriovenous anastomoses of the superficial and deep plexuses (fig. 4). Vascular looping and telangiectatic vessels that would normally be obscured by leakage on FA can be easily visualized. Areas of nonperfused retina on OCTA have been shown to be correlated with areas of ischemic capillary nonperfusion on FA in patients with ischemic BRVO (fig. 4) [19]. As with CRVO, the decrease in vascular perfusion is most prominent in the deep plexus, and the FAZ is more enlarged than normal. This evaluation is important since enlargement of the FAZ in eyes with BRVO may represent macular ischemia and could be an important feature contributing to visual acuity impairment in these eyes [20]. In ischemic BRVO, neovascularization of the optic nerve can occur and is easily detected on OCTA (fig. 5).

Disadvantages of Optical Coherence Tomography Angiography for Retinal Vein Occlusion

In cases in which significant retinal thinning or macular edema causes distortion of the retinal architecture, delineation of the retinal layers for auto-

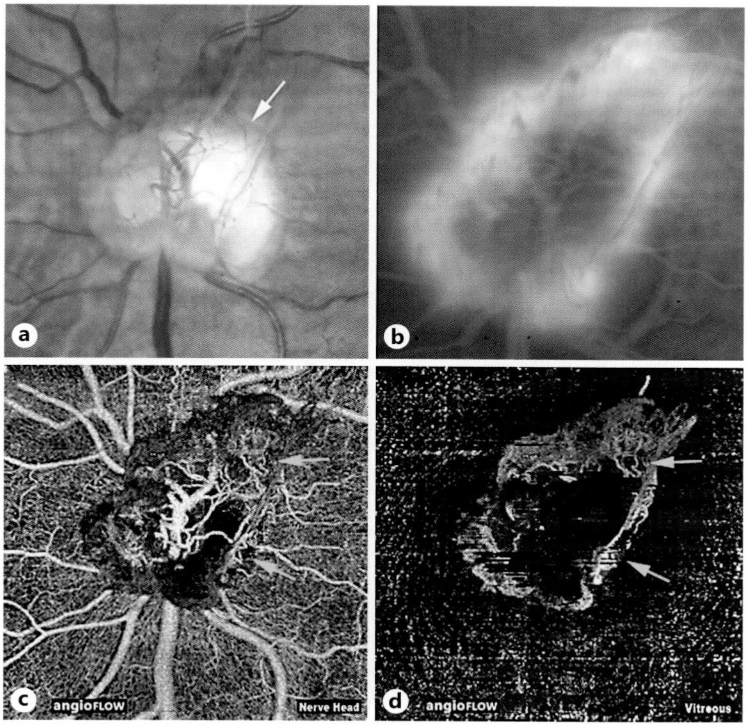

Fig. 5. Sixty-year-old Caucasian male with branch retinal vein occlusion. **a** Color fundus photograph demonstrates neovascularization over the optic nerve (white arrow). **b** Late-late phase fluorescein angiography demonstrates hyperfluorescence of the optic nerve secondary to neovascularization leakage. **c** OCT angiogram of the optic nerve head demonstrates well-delineated fine abnormal vessels (yellow arrow). **d, c** OCT angiogram of the vitreous with detected abnormal flow from neovascular vessels (yellow arrow).

mated segmentation of the superficial and deep retinal capillary plexuses becomes challenging and less accurate. An apparent decrease in vascular perfusion is more prominent in patients with macular edema; however, this may be caused by signal attenuation secondary to a shadowing effect of fluid accumulation or by displacement of vessels by fluid, thereby leading to potential overestimation of the degree of decreased vascular perfusion. In addition, OCTA has a limited field of view, does not allow for visualization of leakage, has an increased potential for artifacts (blink and movement) and cannot detect blood flow below the lowest threshold flow.

Conclusion

Further improvement of OCTA is still required for this imaging modality to have a role in daily clinical application that is comparable to that of FA in many clinical settings. However, there are some obvious advantages of OCTA compared to dye-based angiography for analysis of retinal vascular diseases such as RVO, including rapid and comfortable image acquisition, depth resolution, the lack of a need for invasive dye injection, assessment of the retinal capillary networks at different depths and better quantification of the FAZ area. The absence of information on dynamic blood flow at the capillary level and vascular leakage, which is provided by conventional FA, is its major limitation. However, at this point, with the development of OCTA, OCT as a single modality provides most of the multidimensional information needed to manage patients with vein occlusions. This is because OCTA can now provide both structural and vascular information, in most cases obviating the need for invasive techniques such as dye injection in the investigation and management of patients with vein occlusions.

References

1 Baseline and early natural history report. The central vein occlusion study. Arch Ophthalmol 1993;111:1087–1095.
2 Rehak M, Wiedemann P: Retinal vein thrombosis: pathogenesis and management. J Thromb Haemost 2010;8:1886–1894.
3 Awdeh RM, Elsing SH, Deramo VA, Stinnett S, Lee PP, Fekrat S: Vision-related quality of life in persons with unilateral branch retinal vein occlusion using the 25-item national eye institute visual function questionnaire. Br J Ophthalmol 2010;94:319–323.
4 Coscas G, Loewenstein A, Augustin A, Bandello F, Battaglia Parodi M, Lanzetta P, Mones J, de Smet M, Soubrane G, Staurenghi G: Management of retinal vein occlusion–consensus document. Ophthalmologica 2011;226:4–28.
5 Ha SO, Kim DY, Sohn CH, Lim KS: Anaphylaxis caused by intravenous fluorescein: clinical characteristics and review of literature. Intern Emerg Med 2014;9:325–330.
6 Musa F, Muen WJ, Hancock R, Clark D: Adverse effects of fluorescein angiography in hypertensive and elderly patients. Acta Ophthalmol Scand 2006;84:740–742.
7 Garski TR, Staller BJ, Hepner G, Banka VS, Finney RA Jr: Adverse reactions after administration of indocyanine green. JAMA 1978;240:635.
8 Snodderly DM, Weinhaus RS, Choi JC: Neural-vascular relationships in central retina of macaque monkeys (macaca fascicularis). J Neurosci 1992;12:1169–1193.

9 Sarraf D, Rahimy E, Fawzi AA, Sohn E, Barbazetto I, Zacks DN, Mittra RA, Klancnik JM Jr, Mrejen S, Goldberg NR, Beardsley R, Sorenson JA, Freund KB: Paracentral acute middle maculopathy: a new variant of acute macular neuroretinopathy associated with retinal capillary ischemia. JAMA Ophthalmol 2013;131:1275–1287.
10 Jonathan E, Enfield J, Leahy MJ: Correlation mapping method for generating microcirculation morphology from optical coherence tomography (oct) intensity images. J Biophotonics 2011;4:583–587.
11 An L, Wang RK: In vivo volumetric imaging of vascular perfusion within human retina and choroids with optical micro-angiography. Opt Express 2008;16:11438–11452.
12 Matsunaga D, Yi J, Puliafito CA, Kashani AH: Oct angiography in healthy human subjects. Ophthalmic Surg Lasers Imaging Retina 2014;45:510–515.
13 Kashani AH, Lee SY, Moshfeghi A, Durbin MK, Puliafito CA: Optical coherence tomography angiography of retinal venous occlusion. Retina 2015;35:2323–2331.
14 Ruminski D, Sikorski BL, Bukowska D, Szkulmowski M, Krawiec K, Malukiewicz G, Bieganowski L, Wojtkowski M: Oct angiography by absolute intensity difference applied to normal and diseased human retinas. Biomed Opt Express 2015;6:2738–2754.

15 Rahimy E, Sarraf D, Dollin ML, Pitcher JD, Ho AC: Paracentral acute middle maculopathy in nonischemic central retinal vein occlusion. Am J Ophthalmol 2014;158:372–380.e1.
16 Yu S, Pang CE, Gong Y, Freund KB, Yannuzzi LA, Rahimy E, Lujan BJ, Tabandeh H, Cooney MJ, Sarraf D: The spectrum of superficial and deep capillary ischemia in retinal artery occlusion. Am J Ophthalmol 2015;159:53–63.e1–e2.
17 Mendis KR, Balaratnasingam C, Yu P, Barry CJ, McAllister IL, Cringle SJ, Yu DY: Correlation of histologic and clinical images to determine the diagnostic value of fluorescein angiography for studying retinal capillary detail. Invest Ophthalmol Vis Sci 2010;51:5864–5869.
18 Spaide RF, Klancnik JM Jr, Cooney MJ: Retinal vascular layers imaged by fluorescein angiography and optical coherence tomography angiography. JAMA Ophthalmol 2015;133:45–50.
19 Kuehlewein L, An L, Durbin MK, Sadda SR: Imaging areas of retinal nonperfusion in ischemic branch retinal vein occlusion with swept-source oct microangiography. Ophthalmic Surg Lasers Imaging Retina 2015;46:249–252.
20 Parodi MB, Visintin F, Della Rupe P, Ravalico G: Foveal avascular zone in macular branch retinal vein occlusion. Int Ophthalmol 1995;19:25–28.

Nadia K. Waheed, MD, MPH
New England Eye Center at Tufts Medical Center
260 Tremont Street, Biewend Building, 9–11th Floor
Boston, MA 02116 (USA)
E-Mail nadiakwaheed@gmail.com

Bandello F, Souied EH, Querques G (eds): OCT Angiography in Retinal and Macular Diseases.
Dev Ophthalmol. Basel, Karger, 2016, vol 56, pp 139–145 (DOI: 10.1159/000442806)

Optical Coherence Tomography Angiography of Deep Capillary Ischemia

Julia Nemiroff[a] · Nopasak Phasukkijwatana[a] · David Sarraf[a, b]

[a]Stein Eye Institute, David Geffen School of Medicine at University of California Los Angeles, Los Angeles, Calif., [b]Greater Los Angeles VA Healthcare Center, Los Angeles, Calif., USA

Abstract

Paracentral acute middle maculopathy (PAMM) is defined by the spectral-domain optical coherence tomography (OCT) finding of paracentral hyper-reflective band-like lesions of the inner nuclear layer (INL) of the macula that progress to corresponding areas of severe INL thinning. *En face* analysis has enabled more detailed analyses and quantifications of these lesions and has provided insights into the pathogenesis of this abnormality. While there is a wealth of demographic and anatomical data indicating that these PAMM lesions are the result of an INL infarct, OCT angiography is the first modality to provide direct evidence. Several studies have recently shown that old PAMM lesions are indeed associated with ischemia of the deep capillary retinal plexus, while acute lesions may or may not show initial perfusion of the deep capillary retinal plexus.

© 2016 S. Karger AG, Basel

Paracentral Acute Middle Maculopathy and Deep Retinal Capillary Ischemia

Paracentral acute middle maculopathy (PAMM) is a recently described entity in patients presenting with an acute-onset paracentral scotoma. Spectral-domain optical coherence tomography (SD-OCT) findings include hyper-reflective band-like lesions at the level of the inner nuclear layer (INL). Although these acute lesions resolve, corresponding atrophy of the INL ensues, resulting in a permanent paracentral visual field defect suggestive of an INL infarct. PAMM can be idiopathic, or it can be secondary to a local retinal vascular or systemic disease, such as diabetic retinopathy [1, 2], retinal artery occlusion [2], central retinal vein occlusion [3], sickle cell retinopathy [2], or Purtscher's retinopathy [2], further supporting an ischemic pathogenesis.

It is thought that deep retinal capillary ischemia is the causative factor for the development of these lesions, as the intermediate and deep retinal capillary plexuses (DCP) flank the inner and outer boundaries of the INL, respectively [4–8]. Fluorescein angiography, the reference standard for visualizing the retinal vasculature, has limited depth resolution [9]. With optical coherence tomography angiography (OCTA), it is possible to obtain high resolution, depth-resolved *en face* images of the retinal microvasculature, including the DCP [10].

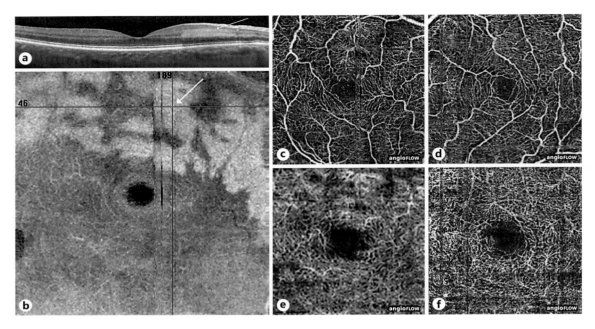

Fig. 1. A 72-year-old hypertensive male presented with a 3-day history of vision loss in his right eye. The best-corrected visual acuity was 20/20 in each eye. Fundus examination showed a subtle patch of retinal whitening in the superior macula of the right eye, and the results of retinal examination of the left eye were normal. An occult branch retinal artery occlusion was suspected. **a** Spectral domain OCT of the hyper-reflective band-like lesion (arrow) consistent with paracentral acute middle maculopahy (PAMM). **b** Three-by-three millimeter en face spectral domain OCT with segmentation of the inner nuclear layer (INL) in the right eye shows characteristic PAMM lesions (white arrow) corresponding to the hyper-reflective, band-like lesions at the level of the INL. Three-by-three millimeter macular cube OCT angiography showing en face projection of the superficial capillary plexus (SCP) (**c, d**) and DCP (**e, f**) of the right and left eyes, respectively. The SCP is normal in each eye, and the DCP is normal in the left eye. The DCP in the affected right eye demonstrates patent perfusion superiorly. Although there are patchy dark areas in the superior aspect of the image, careful inspection demonstrates persistent flow within both the light and dark areas. Note the bright areas of flow corresponding to the PAMM lesions with en face imaging. Vessel density analysis of the 3 × 3 block did not demonstrate any significant difference in capillary density between the right and left eyes (figure adapted from Nemiroff et al. [10]).

Focal Lesions in the Acute Phase

PAMM lesions can be focal (or multifocal) and confined to a segment of the macula, or they can be diffuse, as with central retinal artery occlusion (CRAO). During the acute phase, both lesions appear as hyper-reflective bands in the INL on SD-OCT. Once the hyper-reflective lesions resolve, a legacy of atrophy of the INL remains. Interestingly, OCTA of acute focal lesions may demonstrate patent perfusion of the DCP (fig. 1).

Paracentral Acute Middle Maculopathy and Ischemia-Reperfusion Injury

Preservation of perfusion in these lesions may indicate the existence of an ischemia-reperfusion mechanism, as proposed by 2 recent independent studies [5, 10]. Ischemia-reperfusion injury is a condition in which blood flow returns to a tissue after a period of ischemia. Reperfusion limits immediate retinal damage but is accompanied by mechanisms such as the generation of excessive

Nemiroff · Phasukkijwatana · Sarraf

reactive oxygen species [11], nitric oxide neurotoxicity [12, 13], and inflammation [14]. In rat retinas, ischemia-reperfusion leads to capillary dropout after 8–14 days, and it has been demonstrated that the vessels of the DCP are particularly susceptible to reperfusion injury, as opposed to the vessels of the superficial capillary plexus (SCP) [15]. The pathogenesis of PAMM may be related to ischemia-reperfusion injury under select circumstances, accounting for the persistent capillary flow in some focal acute PAMM lesions and the subsequent legacy of atrophy of the INL associated with loss of the DCP. Two studies conducted by Nemiroff et al. and Sridhar et al. have recently proposed this mechanism.

Diffuse Acute Paracentral Acute Middle Maculopathy Lesions Caused by Central Retinal Artery Occlusion

In the case of diffuse PAMM occurring in the setting of CRAO, i.e. large vessel obstruction, capillary reperfusion may never occur, causing severe acute impairment of flow within the DCP. OCTA of these lesions acutely demonstrate decreased perfusion within the DCP. Imaging of the DCP demonstrates significant projection artifact, or reflection, from the SCP (fig. 2).

Old Paracentral Acute Middle Maculopathy Lesions

The hyper-reflective band-like lesions of the INL characteristic of PAMM in the acute setting eventually resolve over weeks, and corresponding thinning of the INL ensues, indicative of old PAMM lesions or old INL infarcts. OCTA during this chronic phase demonstrates loss of flow within the DCP. Patchy flow voids may be identified within the DCP, and evidence of projection artifacts may be detected from the overlying SCP (fig. 3).

Calculating Vessel Densities of the Superficial and Deep Capillary Plexuses

Vessel density analysis and quantification of the SCP and DCP may be performed using publically available imaging software, such as Fiji ImageJ 2.0.0-rc-29/1.49q (http://fiji.sc/Fiji) [16] and GNU Image Manipulation Program (GIMP) 2.8.14 (http://gimp.org). Fiji is used to binarize (i.e. render images black and white) and skeletonize *en face* images of the SCP and DCP, showing blood vessels as 1-pixel-wide lines. GIMP is used to count the numbers of black pixels and total pixels. Vessel density is then calculated as [(pixels of vessels) (3/304)]/(area in mm^2) in mm^{-1} [17, 18]. In cases with partial or complete projection artifact from the SCP, as seen when there is severe hypoperfusion, Fiji can be used to binarize the SCP and DCP images. GIMP is then used to subtract the black pixels of the SCP from the DCP image. The resulting DCP image is skeletonized using Fiji software, and the number of pixels is calculated using GIMP. Vessel density calculation is then repeated in the manner described above (fig. 4).

Segmentation

Location of segmentation can impact the appearance of the SCP and DCP. In most normal eyes, standard segmentation provides accurate images. The SCP slab can be positioned between the internal limiting membrane (offset 3 μm) and the inner plexiform layer (offset 15 μm). The DCP slab can be positioned between the inner plexiform layer (offset 15 μm) and the outer plexiform layer (offset 70 μm). In cases of severe thinning of the INL, manual segmentation can help to achieve more accurate analysis of the DCP. It is advisable to use a thinner 30-μm band and to manually adjust it to include the DCP.

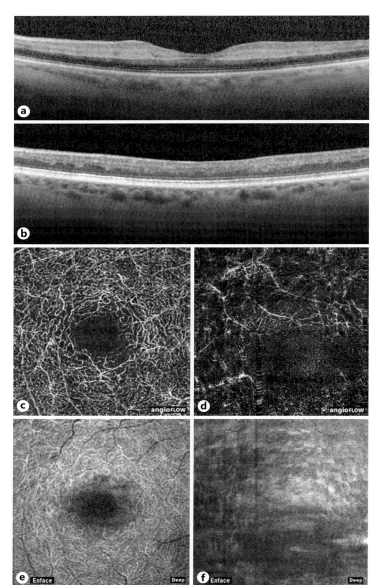

Fig. 2. Central retinal artery occlusion and PAMM of the left eye in an 82-year-old male. **a** Spectral-domain optical coherence tomography (SD-OCT) of the left eye shows band-like hyper-reflective lesions of the INL, consistent with PAMM. **b** SD-OCT of the left eye at 1-year follow-up shows diffuse attenuation of the INL, consistent with old PAMM or a diffuse INL infarct. **c** On 1-year follow-up, 3 × 3 mm macular cube OCTA with *en face* segmentation of the DCP in the right eye shows normal flow. **d** On 1-year follow-up, 3 × 3 mm macular cube OCTA with *en face* segmentation of the DCP in the left eye shows significant loss of flow within the DCP, with some projection artifacts from the SCP, as demonstrated by the identification of larger-caliber vessels of the SCP. **e, f** On 1-year follow-up, *en face* SD-OCT image of the unaffected right eye shows a normal DCP (**e**), but the DCP is completely absent in the affected left eye (**f**) (figure adapted from Nemiroff et al. [10]).

Classification of Paracentral Acute Middle Maculopathy Lesions Based on Optical Coherence Tomography Angiography Appearance

A recent study [5] has proposed a classification scheme for PAMM based on the patterns seen on OCTA and the presumed pathophysiological mechanism. The following three patterns were described: arteriolar, globular, and fern-like. The arteriolar pattern was observed most commonly and showed band-like hyper-reflectivity corresponding to the distribution of a large retinal arteriole, and it is caused by either transient or true arteriolar

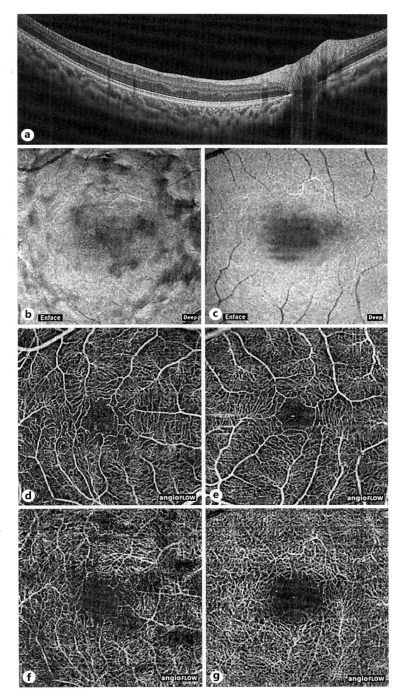

Fig. 3. *En face* OCT angiography and SD-OCT of old PAMM lesions in a 9-year-old boy. **a** SD-OCT images of the right eye show severe thinning of the INL and outer plexiform layer in a patchy parafoveal distribution, consistent with old PAMM lesions, i.e. old INL infarcts. *En face* SD-OCT image of the right eye shows patchy parafoveal loss of the DCP (**b**) in contrast with the normal left eye (**c**). Three-by-three millimeter macular cube OCTA with *en face* projection, capturing the SCP (**d, e**) and DCP (**f, g**) of the right and left eyes, demonstrates patchy parafoveal loss of flow within the DCP in the right eye (**f**) but shows normal flow in the other images (**d, e, g**) (figure adapted from Nemiroff et al. [10]).

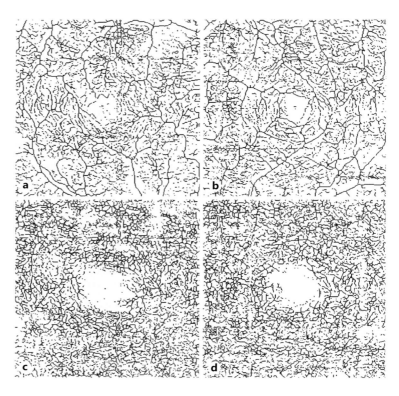

Fig. 4. OCTA scans of the 72-year-old male with multifocal PAMM described in figure 1. Images of the SCP (**a, b**) and DCP (**c, d**) of the right and left eyes, respectively, have been transformed into binary, skeletonized vessel maps using Fiji software to assess the vessel density as the total vessel length per area (mm^{-1}). There was minimal difference in vessel density between each eye in the SCP (12.9 mm^{-1} in normal left eye versus 12.5 mm^{-1} in affected right eye, reduction of –3.1%) and the DCP (17.6 mm^{-1} in normal left eye versus 17.8 mm^{-1} in affected right eye, difference of +0.8%) (figure adapted from Nemiroff et al. [10]).

occlusion. The globular pattern showed either a focal ovoid patch or multifocal ovoid patches of middle retina hyper-reflectivity caused by distal pericapillary or capillary ischemia. The fern-like pattern was seen in the setting of central retinal vein occlusion with multifocal parafoveal middle retina hyper-reflectivity due to perivenular ischemia. A combination of patterns is possible.

Optical Coherence Tomography Angiography Limitations of Deep Capillary Retinal Plexus Imaging in Paracentral Acute Middle Maculopathy

There are some challenges that arise with OCTA of the DCP. Cases of diffuse PAMM associated with CRAO show marked loss of the DCP with overlying projection artifacts from the SCP. To more accurately quantify the vessel density in

these cases, imaging software is required to subtract the vasculature of the SCP from that of the DCP, and the resulting vessel density is calculated. This method of vessel density calculation has been proposed in a recent study [10] but has not been validated, and it likely leads to underestimation of the true plexus, as a portion of the true DCP is removed during processing. A further limitation of OCTA is that it is currently impossible to separate the intermediate capillary plexus from the DCP.

As this imaging field advances, with improved segmentation technology, we may be able to determine whether the intermediate capillary plexus or DCP is more important in the etiology of PAMM.

Further technical limitations include segmentation errors in scans and low quality, which are caused by movement artifacts or retinal pathology, requiring manual segmentation. Motion artifacts can be addressed by including faster eye tracking to improve image quality, especially in subjects with poor fixation and reduced visual acuity. In addition, OCTA can only be used to map vessels with flow, and therefore, it is not possible to definitively state whether flow is absent or is simply too slow to be visualized.

Conclusion

PAMM lesions (i.e. INL infarcts) can be imaged accurately and noninvasively by OCTA, and studies have confirmed associated hypoperfusion of the DCP. The objective vessel density can be calculated to quantify the degree of ischemia. While focal acute PAMM lesions may maintain perfusion, old PAMM lesions develop a corresponding loss of flow within the DCP (and intermediate capillary plexus). Diffuse PAMM lesions occurring in the setting of CRAO lead to severe nonperfusion of the DCP in both acute and chronic cases. Ischemia-reperfusion injury may be responsible for the pathogenesis of some focal PAMM lesions.

References

1 Yu S, Pang CE, Gong Y, et al: The spectrum of superficial and deep capillary ischemia in retinal artery occlusion. Am J Ophthalmol 2015;159:53–63.
2 Chen X, Rahimy E, Sergott RC, et al: Spectrum of retinal vascular diseases associated with paracentral acute middle maculopathy. Am J Ophthalmol 2015;160:26–34.
3 Rahimy E, Sarraf D, Dollin ML, et al: Paracentral acute middle maculopathy in nonischemic central retinal vein occlusion. Am J Ophthalmol 2014;158: 372–380.
4 Sarraf D, Rahimy E, Fawzi AA, et al: Paracentral acute middle maculopathy: a new variant of acute macular neuroretinopathy associated with retinal capillary ischemia. JAMA Ophthalmol 2013; 131:1275–1287.
5 Sridhar J, Shahlaee A, Rahimy E, et al: Optical coherence tomography angiography and en face optical coherence tomography features of paracentral acute middle maculopathy. Am J Ophthalmol 2015;160:1259–1268.
6 Khan MA, Rahimy E, Shahlaee A, et al: En face optical coherence tomography imaging of deep capillary plexus abnormalities in paracentral acute middle maculopathy. Ophthalmic Surg Lasers Imaging Retina 2015;46:972–975.

7 Tsui I, Sarraf D: Paracentral acute middle maculopathy and acute macular neuroretinopathy. Ophthalmic Surg Lasers Imaging Retina 2013;44(6 suppl):S33–S35.
8 Rahimy E, Sarraf D: Paracentral acute middle maculopathy spectral-domain optical coherence tomography feature of deep capillary ischemia. Curr Opin Ophthalmol 2014;25:207–212.
9 Weinhaus RS, Burke JM, Delori FC, et al: Comparison of fluorescein angiography with microvascular anatomy of macaque retinas. Exp Eye Res 1995;61:1–16.
10 Nemiroff J, Kuehlewein L, Rahimy E, et al: Assessing deep retinal capillary ischemia in paracentral acute middle maculopathy by optical coherence tomography angiography. Am J Ophthalmol DOI: 10.1016/j.ajo.2015.10.026.
11 Szabo ME, Droy-Lefaix MT, Doly M, et al: Ischemia and reperfusion-induced histologic changes in the rat retina. Demonstration of a free radical-mediated mechanism. Invest Ophthalmol Vis Sci 1991;32:1471–1478.

12 Hangai M, Yoshimura N, Hiroi K, et al: Inducible nitric oxide synthase in retinal ischemia-reperfusion injury. Exp Eye Res 1996;63:501–509.
13 Neufeld AH, Kawai S, Das S, et al: Loss of retinal ganglion cells following retinal ischemia: the role of inducible nitric oxide synthase. Exp Eye Res 2002;75: 521–528.
14 Tsujikawa A, Ogura Y, Hiroshiba N, et al: Retinal ischemia-reperfusion injury attenuated by blocking of adhesion molecules of vascular endothelium. Invest Ophthalmol Vis Sci 1999;40:1183–1190.
15 Nakahara T, Hoshino M, Hoshino S, et al: Structural and functional changes in retinal vasculature induced by retinal ischemia-reperfusion in rats. Exp Eye Res 2015;135:134–145.
16 Schindelin J, Arganda-Carreras I, Frise E, et al: Fiji: an open-source platform for biological-image analysis. Nat Methods 2012;9:676–682.
17 Tam J, Martin JA, Roorda A: Noninvasive visualization and analysis of parafoveal capillaries in humans. Invest Ophthalmol Vis Sci 2010;51:1691–1698.
18 Zheng D, LaMantia A-S, Purves D: Specialized vascularization of the primate visual cortex. J Neurosci 1991;11:2622–2629.

David Sarraf, MD
Retinal Disorders and Ophthalmic Genetics Division
Stein Eye Institute, David Geffen School of Medicine at UCLA
100 Stein Plaza, Los Angeles, CA 90095 (USA)
E-Mail dsarraf@ucla.edu

Bandello F, Souied EH, Querques G (eds): OCT Angiography in Retinal and Macular Diseases.
Dev Ophthalmol. Basel, Karger, 2016, vol 56, pp 146–158 (DOI: 10.1159/000442807)

Optical Coherence Tomography Angiography of Macular Telangiectasia Type 2

Luiz Roisman[a, b] · Philip J. Rosenfeld[a]

[a]Department of Ophthalmology, Bascom Palmer Eye Institute, University of Miami Miller School of Medicine, Miami, Fla., USA;
[b]Department of Ophthalmology, Federal University of São Paulo, São Paulo, Brazil

Abstract

Macular telangiectasia type 2 (MacTel2) is a disease of the central macula that affects all microvascular layers of the retina and also includes neovascularization arising from both the retinal and choroidal circulations. As a result, MacTel2 is the ideal macular disease for imaging with optical coherence tomography (OCT) angiography (OCTA). In MacTel2, the earliest changes in the retinal microvasculature involve the temporal aspect of the parafoveal deep capillary plexus, and OCTA reveals these changes. Microvascular abnormalities then extend circumferentially around the fovea and into the superficial capillary plexus. As the disease progresses, dilated anastomoses form between the superficial and deep capillary plexuses, and the retina becomes more atrophic, with the formation of cysts and the loss of photoreceptor outer segments. In some patients, the anastomoses between the plexuses progress to subretinal neovascularization, with connections to the choroidal vasculature. OCTA provides clear advantages over current imaging modalities, such as traditional OCT imaging, reflectance fundus imaging, autofluorescence imaging, fluorescein angiography, and indocyanine green angiography, for MacTel2 because it is safer, cheaper, more comfortable for the patient, and more easily repeatable, it can be performed during follow-up visits, and it produces both intensity-based OCT images and flow-based images, which allow for visualization of the macular microvasculature. OCTA is the only imaging modality needed for the diagnosis and monitoring of MacTel2 at every stage of disease progression.

© 2016 S. Karger AG, Basel

In 1982, Gass and Oyakawa [1] were the first to identify forms of retinal telangiectasia limited to the parafoveal region that were not associated with any other known disease. They named this

Précis
Angiography with swept-source optical coherence tomography; characterization of macular telangiectasia in its different stages.

condition idiopathic juxtafoveolar retinal telangiectasia and classified it into four groups. Over the years, different classifications have been created for this condition, [1, 2] and in 2006, Yannuzzi et al. [3] simplified the classification into the following two groups: aneurysmal telangiectasia or idiopathic macular telangiectasia type 1 and perifoveal telangiectasia, also known as idiopathic macular telangiectasia type 2 (MacTel2). Eyes with MacTel2 are subdivided into a nonproliferative stage, characterized by telangiectasia and foveal atrophy, and a proliferative stage, characterized by the presence of subretinal neovascularization (SNV) [3].

MacTel2 is an acquired condition that most commonly affects middle-aged patients, with a mean age of 55 years. Males and females are affected equally. It is a bilateral, asymmetric disorder that can appear unilateral in its early stages [2, 3]. Initially, patients are generally asymptomatic. The only biomicroscopic finding might be a slight loss of retinal transparency with a grayish coloration, usually localized to the temporal juxtafoveolar area. The grayish-appearing area of the temporal parafoveolar retina enlarges to approximately one disc diameter in size [1–4]. With progression of the disease, telangiectatic changes occur within the temporal juxtafoveal microvasculature. Patients may experience nonspecific symptoms, such as the blurring of vision, a paracentral or central scotoma, difficulty with reading, and metamorphopsia [5]. Typically in MacTel2, slightly dilated and blunted retinal vessels in the temporal parafoveal retina appear to form right angles and travel toward the outer retina. Multiple, crystalline, golden, tiny, refractile deposits near the telangiectasias are a common finding and occur in about 45% of eyes [1, 2, 6]. Stellate foci of intraretinal pigmented plaques composed of hyperplastic retinal pigment epithelium (RPE) cells may develop along the right-angle vessels. There is not usually lipid exudation or hemorrhages associated with MacTel2 unless SNV is present [2]. During the proliferative phase, patients may complain of vision loss, and signs of SNV may be found, such as subretinal hemorrhage, macular edema, and hard exudates [3].

The cause of MacTel2 remains elusive, but our understanding of the disease is progressing due to advances in macular imaging. The gold standard for the diagnosis of MacTel2 is fluorescein angiography (FA). Typically, the perifoveal capillaries are dilated, with leakage in the parafoveal temporal area [2]. FA may also demonstrate right-angle vessels, and intraretinal and/or subretinal anastomoses may originate from these vessels [3]. When present, SNV appears to originate from the deep retinal circulation and is characterized by early and late fluorescein leakage, but the presence of SNV may be difficult to visualize due to the overlying fluorescein leakage from the abnormal retinal vasculature [3, 7]. Routine optical coherence tomography (OCT) imaging can be performed to identify the increased retinal thickness that accompanies SNV; however, it is never seen in the absence of SNV, even though fluorescein leakage is a common finding in this disease.

Another useful imaging modality is fundus autofluorescence (AF), using an excitation wavelength of 488 nm. Normal eyes show central foveal masking on AF due to the central accumulation of macular pigment. A reduced macular pigment density or and/or changes in its topographic distribution may affect this masking. In the absence of RPE atrophy, areas of Mueller cell and photoreceptor atrophy have reduced pigment densities, and these areas with reduced pigment densities show increased AF intensities relative to surrounding areas with healthy Mueller cells and photoreceptors [8, 9]. These areas of relatively increased autofluorescence are first detected in the temporal parafoveal region. Hyporeflective cavities in the neurosensory retina are also associated with these relative increases in AF signal, and they may further be explained by reduced absorption of excitation light by photoreceptors and/or macular pigment [10]. Thus, the increased AF signal is most likely due to the depletion of luteal pigment rather than to increased lipofuscin accumulation in the RPE [11].

OCT has become a valuable tool for diagnosing and studying MacTel2. Unlike other retinal vascular disorders, such as diabetic macular edema and branch retinal vein occlusion, intraretinal hyporeflective spaces and macular leakage on FA are not associated with increased retinal thickening [12, 13]. Important changes on OCT imaging may include hyporeflective cavities within the inner retina, and they are usually located in the foveal pit, with a predilection for the temporal slope. At the foveola, an inner lamellar cyst appears as tissue is lost [3], with the internal limiting membrane spanning across it or draping over it. This unique feature is called an internal limiting membrane drape [13]. Abnormalities along the inner segment/outer segment/ellipsoid (IS/OS/E) zone are closely related to the loss of retinal sensitivity. Thus, as demonstrated in numerous retinal diseases including MacTel2, there is value in correlating the integrity of the OCT band #2 (the IS/OS/E line) with photoreceptor integrity as a predictor of retinal function [14–17]. With disease progression, atrophy of the outer neurosensory retina becomes increasingly prevalent, with subsequent collapse leading to apposition of the inner retinal layers onto the RPE. Hyperreflective intraretinal lesions are usually associated with pigment plaques, and larger lesions may present as flat hyperreflective structures within the inner retinal layer. Secondary SNV typically presents with macular thickening due to intra- and/or subretinal fluid, and this type of SNV is located in or external to the outer neurosensory retinal layers. Some of the other changes mentioned above, such as foveal cyst formation, intraretinal RPE hyperplasia, foveal atrophy, and absence of edema, are consistent with the hypothesis of progressive retinal tissue loss, most likely due to degeneration of Mueller cells and photoreceptors [18, 19].

In recent years, confocal reflectance imaging using a confocal scanning laser ophthalmoscope (HRA2, Heidelberg Engineering, Heidelberg, Germany) has emerged as a very sensitive and noninvasive method for the diagnosis of MacTel2, as well as for the monitoring of its progression and for its differentiation from other conditions [20, 21]. Confocal blue reflectance imaging (at 488 nm) is particularly helpful in the diagnosis of the early disease stages, which are the most difficult to detect clinically. Confocal blue reflectance imaging discloses a well-defined, generally oval parafoveal area of increased reflectance that corresponds to, but is slightly larger than, the area of leakage on late-phase angiography [20, 21]. Confocal infrared reflectance (at 820 nm), on the other hand, is helpful for monitoring progression, showing uniformly increased reflectance corresponding to the area of leakage on angiography during the early stages, and detecting pigment clumping or SNV, corresponding to decreased reflectance in the area of leakage, during the late stages [21].

Since microperimetry seems to be the most appropriate test for measuring functional deficits in patients with MacTel2, several studies have reported structural/functional correlations based on microperimetry data [8, 17, 22, 23]. Structural damage to the outer retinal photoreceptor layers has been associated with a loss of retinal sensitivity, as detected by microperimetry, but structural changes limited to the inner retina and macular thickness have been shown to have no correlation with sensitivity loss. The presence of pigment hypertrophy and blunted venules has been shown to have the most significant associations with decreased visual acuity [23, 24].

With the development of optical coherence tomography angiography (OCTA), it is now possible to noninvasively image the retinal and choroidal microvasculature without the use of exogenous intravenous dye injection. Moreover, routine anatomic intensity-based OCT images are also obtained as part of the OCTA scanning strategy. OCTA has the typical advantages of OCT imaging, including the ability to diagnose MacTel2 and monitor its progression, in addition to the ability to identify abnormal microvasculature in the perifoveal region and to correlate this abnormal microvasculature seen on *en face* OCTA images with leakage seen on FA images, helping to confirm the diagnosis. In addition to being a noninvasive diagnostic strategy, OCTA has the following advantages over FA: it is faster, cheaper, safer, easily repeatable, provides superior image quality, is less affected by the fluorescein leakage that obscures the microvasculature, and provides better imaging through cataracts and segmentation of the retinal and choroidal layers in three dimensions so that the disease process can be better localized. Using this ability to extract and visualize the retinal and choroidal layers in three dimensions, we found that OCTA imaging not only helps to facilitate the early diagnosis of MacTel2 but also provides a better understanding of disease progression and treatment efficacy. It remains to be seen whether the ability to detect leakage on FA provides any diagnostic advantage over OCTA in the early diagnosis of MacTel2 or whether the better visualization of the retinal microvasculature by OCTA due to the absence of leakage provides a superior diagnostic advantage. However, it is clear is that once MacTel2 is diagnosed, OCTA is clearly the superior imaging strategy for documenting disease progression at follow-up.

The central macular microvasculature can be better visualized using OCTA compared with FA imaging [25]. In addition, the lack of leakage can be an advantage in some cases since visualization of the juxtafoveal microvasculature with OCTA is better in the absence of leakage. Further, luteal pigment attenuates the excitation of fluorescein in the central macular region at a 488 nm excitation wavelength, and this attenuation obscures the parafoveal microvasculature. However, this luteal pigment has no effect on OCTA imaging since the central wavelength of the light source used in OCTA is in the near-infrared region (840 nm). Thorell et al. [25] identified some characteristic features of MacTel2 in patients with different stages of the disease using an algorithm known as

optical coherence tomography microangiography (OMAG). Based on this initial study, it appeared as though MacTel2 was the ideal disease for imaging with OMAG-based OCTA because most of the early pathology is contained within the central macula, and the microvascular changes occur within the deep temporal capillary plexus of the retina. As the disease progresses, all central retinal microvasculature layers are involved. Moreover, the microvasculature is better visualized with OCTA than with FA, and OCTA provides better visualization of SNV than FA due to the lack of fluorescein leakage. Further, OCTA is faster, cheaper, and noninvasive, with none of the nausea or anaphylactic risks associated with FA and indocyanine green angiography (ICGA).

While several groups have published spectral domain OCTA images of MacTel2 [26–28], the first published OCTA images of MacTel2 and the best OCTA images of MacTel2 to date have been produced using the OMAG algorithm, with scans performed on a Zeiss 1,050 nm swept-source optical coherence tomography (SS-OCT) prototype [25, 29]. These images are shown in this chapter and were obtained using a scan pattern that was centered on the fovea in a 3 × 3 mm area on the retina. In the transverse scanning direction, a single B-scan was composed of 300 A-scans. Four consecutive B-scans were performed at each fixed location before proceeding to the next transverse position on the retina. A total of 300 B-scan positions located 10 μm apart over a 3-mm distance were performed. The time difference between two successive B-scans was roughly 3.8 ms, which corresponded to a B-scan acquisition rate of 263 B-scans per second. The images of microvascular networks shown herein were obtained using the previously published OMAG algorithm, and in all cases, an intensity differentiation algorithm was applied to extract *in vivo* blood flow information [25, 30, 31]. In these images, the microvasculature from the superficial capillary plexus in the inner retina is colored red, that from the deep capillary plexus is colored green, and any micro-

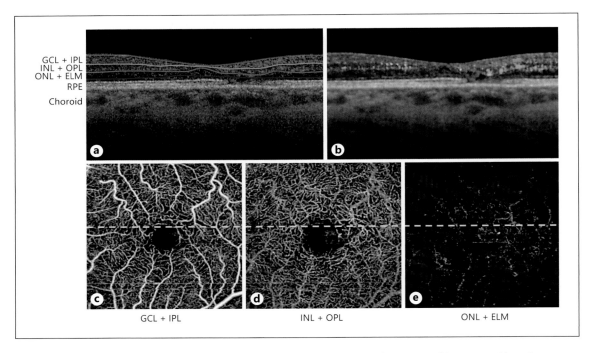

GCL + IPL INL + OPL ONL + ELM RPE Choroid

GCL + IPL   INL + OPL   ONL + ELM

Fig. 1. Optical coherence tomography microangiography (OMAG) images of a 55-year-old woman with early nonproliferative macular telangiectasia type 2 (MacTel2). **a** Horizontal central B-scan with the three layers of retinal segmentation: the inner retinal layer from the ganglion cell layer (GCL) to the inner plexiform layer (IPL), the middle retinal layer from the inner nuclear layer (INL) to the outer plexiform layer (OPL), and the outer retinal layer (ORL) from the outer nuclear layer (ONL) to the external limiting membrane (ELM) layer. **b** Horizontal central B-scan shows the microvascular flow, with the different colors corresponding to the different segmented layers of the retina. **c** *En face* OMAG image from the GCL to the IPL shows no obvious microvascular abnormality. **d** *En face* OMAG image from the INL to the OPL shows subtle alterations in the temporal juxtafoveal microvasculature. **e** *En face* OMAG image from the ONL to the ELM shows a lack of obvious microvasculature. This figure was previously published (courtesy of Dr. Thorell and Dr. Rosenfeld) [25].

vascular structures with flow in the outer retina are colored blue. Averaged OCT B-scans are also provided in the usual manner by showing both cross-sectional B-scans and *en face* images based on just the intensity signals. Thus, with OCTA, we get both intensity images and flow images from the same dataset.

In early nonproliferative MacTel2, two-dimensional OMAG *en face* images usually demonstrate dilated vessels in the deep retinal capillary plexus from the middle retinal layer that are the most pronounced in the region temporal to the fovea. However, no visible alterations in the mi-

crovasculature are found in the superficial vasculature. The OCT B-scan and flow images also show that these dilated vessels are associated with disruption of the IS/OS/E region. The color-coded OMAG images illustrate the area corresponding to the subtle telangiectatic alterations, which is located in the middle retinal layer and is depicted as the prominent green vessel in the temporal juxtafoveal region [25] (fig. 1, 2).

In intermediate, nonproliferative MacTel2, OMAG images show multiple, telangiectatic, microaneurysmal-like dilated vessels residing within the middle retinal layer and extending to the

Fig. 2. OMAG and fluorescein angiography (FA) images of the same patient shown in figure 1. **a** Early-phase FA image shows hyperfluorescence in the temporal juxtafoveal region. **b** Late-phase FA image shows increased hyperfluorescence and leakage. **c** Magnified early-stage FA image shows a detailed view of the hyperfluorescent area that represents the telangiectatic microvasculature. **d** Composite *en face* color-coded OMAG image demonstrates abnormal microvasculature in the middle layers (green). This figure was previously published (courtesy of Dr. Thorell and Dr. Rosenfeld) [25].

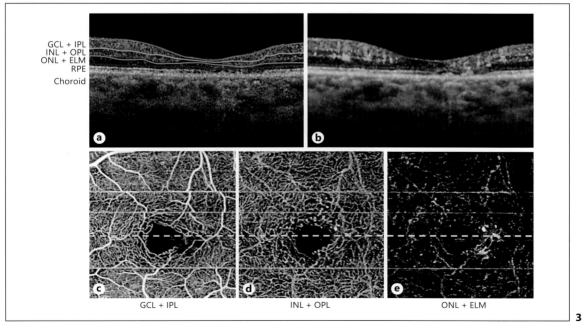

Early-stage FA

Late-stage FA

Magnified early-stage FA

GCL-ELM color

GCL + IPL
INL + OPL
ONL + ELM
RPE
Choroid

GCL + IPL

INL + OPL

ONL + ELM

3

(For legend see next page.)

Fig. 3. OMAG images of a 70-year-old woman with intermediate, nonproliferative MacTel2. **a** Horizontal central B-scan with the three layers of retinal segmentation: the inner retinal layer (GCL + IPL), the middle retinal layer (INL + OPL), and the ORL (ONL + ELM). **b** Horizontal central B-scan shows the microvascular flow, with the different colors corresponding to the different segmented layers of the retina with areas of disruption of the inner segment/outer segment/ ellipsoid region. **c** *En face* OMAG image from the GCL to the IPL shows irregular vessels and vascular dropout in the temporal juxtafoveal region. **d** *En face* OMAG image from the INL to the OPL shows microvascular abnormalities in the perifoveal region. **e** *En face* OMAG image from the ONL to the ELM shows extension of the abnormal microvasculature to the outer retina. This figure was previously published (courtesy of Dr. Thorell and Dr. Rosenfeld) [25].

inner and outer retina, and the outer retinal changes correspond to disruption of the IS/OS/E region [25] (fig. 3, 4).

In late proliferative or neovascular MacTel2, SS-OCTA shows significant alterations in the juxtafoveal capillary network with prominent anastomoses. The presence of abnormal vessels corresponds to an area with retinal vascular anastomoses that extends to the outer retina where the IS/OS/E is disrupted, forming a subretinal fibrovascular plaque (fig. 5–8) [25, 29]. The retinal microvasculature and SNV are visualized better with OCTA using the OMAG algorithm than with FA imaging, and visualization using OCTA is comparable to or better than that obtained with ICGA (fig. 8) [25]. Previously, SNV was thought to arise

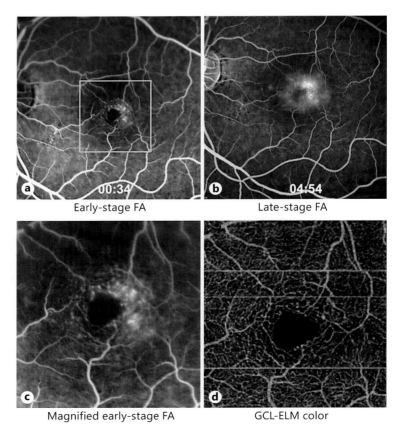

Fig. 4. OMAG and FA images of the same patient as in figure 3. **a** Early-phase FA image shows temporal juxtafoveal hyperfluorescence. **b** Late-phase FA image shows increased hyperfluorescence and leakage. **c** Magnified early-stage FA image shows a detailed view of the hyperfluorescent area that corresponds to the telangiectatic microvasculature. **d** Composite *en face* color-coded OMAG image demonstrates abnormal microvasculature in the middle layers (green), corresponding to the telangiectatic vessels seen on FA imaging in the temporal juxtafoveal location. This figure was previously published (courtesy of Dr. Thorell and Dr. Rosenfeld) [25].

Early-stage FA

Late-stage FA

Magnified early-stage FA

GCL-ELM color

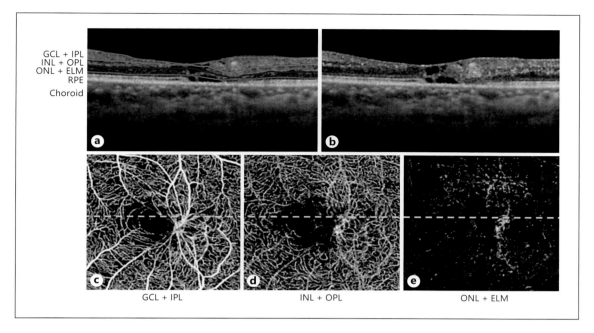

Fig. 5. OMAG images of a 54-year-old woman with late proliferative MacTel2. **a** Horizontal central B-scan with the three layers of retinal segmentation: the inner retinal layer (GCL + IPL), the middle retinal layer (INL + OPL), and the ORL (ONL + ELM). **b** Horizontal central B-scan shows the microvascular flow, with the different colors corresponding to the different segmented layers of the retina. Prominent abnormal flow is observed temporally in the middle and deep retinal layers. Disruption of the inner segment/outer segment/ellipsoid region and retinal cavitation are present. **c** *En face* OMAG image from the GCL to the IPL shows retinal vascular anastomoses in the temporal juxtafoveal region with distortion of the capillary plexus. **d** *En face* OMAG image from the INL to the OPL shows microvascular abnormalities. **e** *En face* OMAG image from the ONL to the ELM shows evidence of the same microvascular alterations extending from the inner and middle retinal layers. This figure was previously published (courtesy of Dr. Thorell and Dr. Rosenfeld) [25].

solely from retinal circulation, but with both ICGA and SS-OCTA, it has become evident that the neovascular complex communicates with both retinal and choroidal circulation. It is unclear at what point the choroidal microvasculature becomes involved with these subretinal neovascular complexes. While retinal anastomoses appear to play a prominent role in establishing SNV, it may be that these neovascular lesions only start to cause exudation-induced vision loss once the choroidal circulation contributes to the lesion [28].

OMAG also demonstrated that the calibers of the retinal vessels and their anastomoses decreased after anti-vascular endothelial growth factor (VEGF) therapy and that the microaneurysmal changes associated with the telangiectatic vessels were not detectable. It remains to be determined whether anti-VEGF therapy actually causes regression of these lesions or whether the blood flow within them is diminished beyond the level of detection (fig. 9) [25, 29]. Since SS-OCTA can be repeated frequently, it is particularly useful for following patients undergoing anti-VEGF therapy.

In summary, MacTel2 is a disease of the central macula that is ideal for imaging with OCTA. It affects all microvascular layers of the retina and also includes retinal and choroidal neovascularization. In MacTel2, OCTA reveals the earliest changes in the temporal parafoveal deep

Fig. 6. OMAG and FA images of the same patient as in figure 5. **a** Early-phase FA shows hyperfluorescence in the temporal juxtafoveal region. **b** Late-phase FA shows leakage in the corresponding area. **c** Magnified early-stage FA image shows a detailed view of the hyperfluorescent area with microvascular abnormalities. **d** Composite *en face* color-coded OMAG image demonstrates abnormal microvascular flow characteristics that correspond to the abnormal microvascular area with leakage seen on FA imaging. This figure was previously published (courtesy of Dr. Thorell and Dr. Rosenfeld) [25].

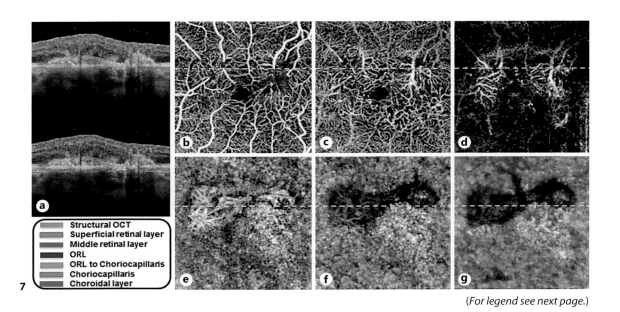

Early-stage FA

Late-stage FA

Magnified early-stage FA

GCL-ELM color

Structural OCT
Superficial retinal layer
Middle retinal layer
ORL
ORL to Choriocapillaris
Choriocapillaris
Choroidal layer

7

(For legend see next page.)

Fig. 7. OMAG images of a 51-year-old woman with late proliferative MacTel2. **a** Horizontal B-scan averaged from four repeated B-scans with and without color-coded blood flow information. The layer and the corresponding color code are shown in the legend. The dotted yellow line in (**b–g**) represents the location of the B-scan. Although vascular leakage cannot be detected by optical coherence tomography (OCT) angiography, the increase in retinal thickness and macular fluid seen on the cross-sectional B-scan images in figure 1a suggest the presence of neovascular leakage. **b–d** Horizontal central B-scan with the three layers of retinal segmentation: the inner retinal layer (GCL + IPL), the middle retinal layer (INL + OPL), and the ORL (ONL + ELM). These overlying retinal layers show circumferential microvascular dropout around the fovea, with prominent anastomoses between the superficial and deep retinal vascular plexuses. **b** *En face* OMAG image from the GCL to the IPL shows abnormally dilated microvasculature in the temporal juxtafoveal region. **c** *En face* OMAG image from the INL to the OPL shows extensive microvascular alterations throughout the juxtafoveal region (**d**). *En face* OMAG image from the ONL to the ELM shows a plaque with abnormal microvascular flow in the outer retina that corresponds to subretinal neovascularization (**e, f**). For better visualization of the subretinal neovascular complex, the segmentation was changed, and three additional layers were created representing a slab from the ORL to the choriocapillaris (CC), which is about 8 μm beneath the Bruch membrane layer; a slab from 8 to 20 μm beneath the Bruch membrane, which includes the CC and inner choroid; and a slab encompassing the choroidal layers beneath the CC to the boundary of the sclera (**e**). *En face* OCT flow image from the ORL to the CC, showing the subretinal neovascular complex. **f** *En face* OCT flow image from the CC. **g** *En face* OCT flow image from the remaining choroidal vasculature. This figure was previously published (courtesy of Dr. Zhang) [29].

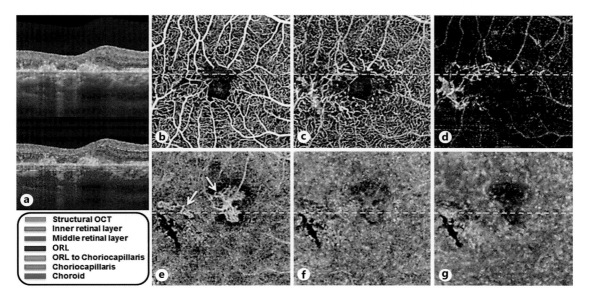

Fig. 8. OMAG images of a 56-year-old man with neovascular MacTel2. **a** Horizontal B-scan averaged from four repeated B-scans with and without color-coded blood flow information. The layer and the corresponding color code are shown in the legend. The dotted yellow line in B–G represents the location of the B-scan. **b** *En face* OCT flow image of the superficial retinal layer. **c** *En face* OCT flow image of the middle retinal layer shows microvascular abnormalities. **d** *En face* OCT flow image of the ORL. **e** *En face* OCT flow image from the ORL to the CC. The white arrows point to choroidal vessels communicating with the subretinal neovascular complex. **f** *En face* OCT flow image from the CC. **g** *En face* flow image from the remaining choroidal vasculature. This figure was previously published (courtesy of Dr. Zhang) [29].

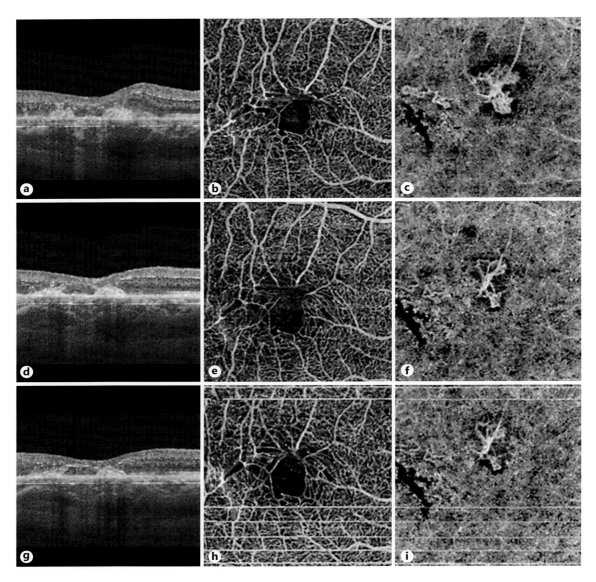

Fig. 9. Comparison of OCT B-scans and OMAG flow images of the patient shown in figure 7 after administration of monthly intravitreal injections of bevacizumab. **a**, **d**, **g** Baseline, 1 month after first injection of bevacizumab and 1 month after second injection of bevacizumab: horizontal B-scan averaged from four repeated B-scans, with color-coded blood flow information showing flattening of the retina and less subretinal flow (pink). **b**, **e**, **h** Baseline, 1 month after first injection of bevacizumab and 1 month after second injection of bevacizumab: composite, color-coded *en face* OCT flow image of the retina, presenting decreasing of the flow in the subretinal neovascular network (blue color for subretinal flow). **c**, **f**, **i** Baseline, 1 month after first injection of bevacizumab and 1 month after second injection of bevacizumab: *En face* OCT flow image from the layer between the outer retina to the inner CC, showing shrinking of the neovascular complex. This figure was previously published (courtesy of Dr. Zhang) [29].

capillary plexus, and these abnormalities then extend circumferentially around the fovea and into the superficial capillary plexus. As the disease progresses, prominent dilated anastomoses form between the superficial and deep capillary plexuses, and SNV can develop and communicate with the choroidal circulation. Overall, SS-OCTA is superior to multimodal imaging using different reflectance techniques, autofluorescence, FA and ICGA for use in the diagnosis and monitoring of MacTel2 because OCTA is fast, comfortable for the patient, safe, less costly, and provides traditional OCT intensity-based imaging along with flow-based imaging that beauti-

References

1 Gass JD, Oyakawa RT: Idiopathic juxtafoveolar retinal telangiectasis. Arch Ophthalmol 1982;100:769–780.

2 Gass JD, Blodi BA: Idiopathic juxtafoveolar retinal telangiectasis. Update of classification and follow-up study. Ophthalmology 1993;100:1536–1546.

3 Yannuzzi LA, Bardal AM, Freund KB, Chen KJ, Eandi CM, Blodi B: Idiopathic macular telangiectasia. Arch Ophthalmol 2006;124:450–460.

4 Mansour AM, Schachat A: Foveal avascular zone in idiopathic juxtafoveolar telangiectasia. Ophthalmologica 1993; 207:9–12.

5 Charbel Issa P, Holz FG, Scholl HP: Metamorphopsia in patients with macular telangiectasia type 2. Doc Ophthalmol 2009;119:133–140.

6 Abujamra S, Bonanomi MT, Cresta FB, Machado CG, Pimentel SL, Caramelli CB: Idiopathic juxtafoveolar retinal telangiectasis: clinical pattern in 19 cases. Ophthalmologica 2000;214:406–411.

7 Soheilian M, Tavallali A, Peyman GA: Identification of intraretinal neovascularization by high-speed indocyanine green angiography in idiopathic perifoveal telangiectasia. Ophthalmic Surg Lasers Imaging 2007;38:167–169.

8 Wong WT, Forooghian F, Majumdar Z, Bonner RF, Cunningham D, Chew EY: Fundus autofluorescence in type 2 idiopathic macular telangiectasia: correlation with optical coherence tomography and microperimetry. Am J Ophthalmol 2009;148:573–583.

9 Zeimer MB, Padge B, Heimes B, Pauleikhoff D: Idiopathic macular telangiectasia type 2:distribution of macular pigment and functional investigations. Retina 2010;30:586–595.

10 Bottoni F, Eandi CM, Pedenovi S, Staurenghi G: Integrated clinical evaluation of Type 2A idiopathic juxtafoveolar retinal telangiectasis. Retina 2010;30:317–326.

11 Gass JD: Muller cell cone, an overlooked part of the anatomy of the fovea centralis: hypotheses concerning its role in the pathogenesis of macular hole and foveomacualr retinoschisis. Arch Ophthalmol 1999;117:821–823.

12 Surguch V, Gamulescu MA, Gabel VP: Optical coherence tomography findings in idiopathic juxtafoveal retinal telangiectasis. Graefes Arch Clin Exp Ophthalmol 2007;245:783–788.

13 Paunescu LA, Ko TH, Duker JS, Chan A, Drexler W, Schuman JS, et al: Idiopathic juxtafoveal retinal telangiectasis: new findings by ultrahigh-resolution optical coherence tomography. Ophthalmology 2006;113:48–57.

14 Sallo FB, Peto T, Egan C, Wolf-Schnurrbusch UE, Clemons TE, Gillies MC, et al: 'En face' OCT imaging of the IS/OS junction line in type 2 idiopathic macular telangiectasia. Invest Ophthalmol Vis Sci 2012;53:6145–6152.

15 Sallo FB, Peto T, Egan C, Wolf-Schnurrbusch UE, Clemons TE, Gillies MC, et al: The IS/OS junction layer in the natural history of type 2 idiopathic macular telangiectasia. Invest Ophthalmol Vis Sci 2012;53:7889–7895.

16 Sallo FB, Leung I, Clemons TE, Peto T, Bird AC, Pauleikhoff D: Multimodal imaging in type 2 idiopathic macular telangiectasia. Retina 2015;35:742–749.

17 Maruko I, Iida T, Sekiryu T, Fujiwara T: Early morphological changes and functional abnormalities in group 2A idiopathic juxtafoveolar retinal telangiectasis using spectral domain optical coherence tomography and microperimetry. Br J Ophthalmol 2008;92:1488–1491.

18 Cohen SM, Cohen ML, El-Jabali F, Pautler SE: Optical coherence tomography findings in nonproliferative group 2a idiopathic juxtafoveal retinal telangiectasis. Retina 2007;27:59–66.

19 Gass JD: Histopathologic study of presumed parafoveal telangiectasis. Retina 2000;20:226–227.

20 Charbel Issa P, Berendschot TT, Staurenghi G, Holz FG, Scholl HP: Confocal blue reflectance imaging in type 2 idiopathic macular telangiectasia. Invest Ophthalmol Vis Sci 2008;49:1172–1177.

21 Charbel Issa P, Finger RP, Helb HM, Holz FG, Scholl HP: A new diagnostic approach in patients with type 2 macular telangiectasia: confocal reflectance imaging. Acta Ophthalmol 2008;86:464–465.

22 Charbel Issa P, Helb HM, Holz FG, Scholl HP, MacTel Study Group: Correlation of macular function with retinal thickness in nonproliferative type 2 idiopathic macular telangiectasia. Am J Ophthalmol 2008;145:169–175.

23 Charbel Issa P, Helb HM, Rohrschneider K, Holz FG, Scholl HP: Microperimetric assessment of patients with type 2 idiopathic macular telangiectasia. Invest Ophthalmol Vis Sci 2007;48:3788–3795.

24 Clemons TE, Gillies MC, Chew EY, Bird AC, Peto T, Figueroa MJ, et al: Baseline characteristics of participants in the natural history study of macular telangiectasia (MacTel) MacTel Project Report No. 2. Ophthalmic Epidemiol 2010;17: 66–73.

25 Thorell MR, Zhang Q, Huang Y, An L, Durbin MK, Laron M, et al: Swept-source OCT angiography of macular telangiectasia type 2. Ophthalmic Surg Lasers Imaging Retina 2014;45:369–380.

26 Zeimer M, Gutfleisch M, Heimes B, Spital G, Lommatzsch A, Pauleikhoff D: Association between changes in macular vasculature in optical coherence tomography- and fluorescein- angiography and distribution of macular pigment in type 2 idiopathic macular telangiectasia. Retina 2015;35:2307–2316.

27 Spaide RF, Klancnik JM Jr, Cooney MJ: Retinal vascular layers in macular telangiectasia type 2 imaged by optical coherence tomographic angiography. JAMA Ophthalmol 2015;133:66–73.

28 Spaide RF, Klancnik JM Jr, Cooney MJ, Yannuzzi LA, Balaratnasingam C, Dansingani KK, et al: Volume-rendering optical coherence tomography angiography of macular telangiectasia type 2. Ophthalmology 2015;122:2261–2269.

29 Zhang Q, Wang RK, Chen CL, Legarreta AD, Durbin MK, An L, et al: Swept source optical coherence tomography angiography of neovascular macular telangiectasia type 2. Retina 2015;35: 2285–2299.

30 Wang RK: Three-dimensional optical micro-angiography maps directional blood perfusion deep within microcirculation tissue beds in vivo. Phys Med Biol 2007;52:N531–N537.

31 Wang RK, Jacques SL, Ma Z, Hurst S, Hanson SR, Gruber A: Three dimensional optical angiography. Opt Express 2007;15:4083–4097.

Philip J. Rosenfeld, MD, PhD
Bascom Palmer Eye Institute
900 NW 17th street
Miami, FL 33136 (USA)
E-Mail prosenfeld@miami.edu

Bandello F, Souied EH, Querques G (eds): OCT Angiography in Retinal and Macular Diseases.
Dev Ophthalmol. Basel, Karger, 2016, vol 56, pp 159–165 (DOI: 10.1159/000442808)

Optical Coherence Tomography Angiography in Dystrophies

Maurizio Battaglia Parodi · Luisa Pierro · Marco Gagliardi · Rosangela Lattanzio ·
Giuseppe Querques · Francesco Bandello

Department of Ophthalmology, Ospedale San Raffaele, Vita-Salute University, Milan, Italy

Abstract

Optical coherence tomography (OCT) angiography (OCT-A) represents an innovative imaging technique which can delineate the retinal and choroidal vascular networks. OCT-A in the assessment of chorio-retinal dystrophies reveal alterations especially located at the level of the deep capillary plexus and the choriocapillaris. This information can have a direct implication on the understanding of the pathogenesis of dystrophies and for their future therapeutic management.

© 2016 S. Karger AG, Basel

Introduction

Optical coherence tomography (OCT) angiography (OCT-A) is an innovative imaging technique based on the highly efficient split-spectrum amplitude-decorrelation angiography algorithm, and it is a valid alternative to conventional angiography [1–3]. OCT-A has several advantages, including the capacity for 3D visualization of retinal and choroidal circulation, noninvasiveness, and rapidity of examination. OCT-A can be virtually exploited for any kind of retino-choroidal disorder to obtain information regarding the characteristic alterations in flow directly 'in vivo'. The application of OCT-A to assess chorioretinal dystrophies has not yet been thoroughly analyzed, although it shows promise for detecting vascular abnormalities, which could be useful for gaining deeper knowledge of both the pathogenesis of dystrophies and their therapeutic implications.

Methods

In this study, OCT-A was performed using a Swept-Source DRI OCT Triton (Topcon Corporation, Japan). Images were analyzed using the Topcon full-spectrum

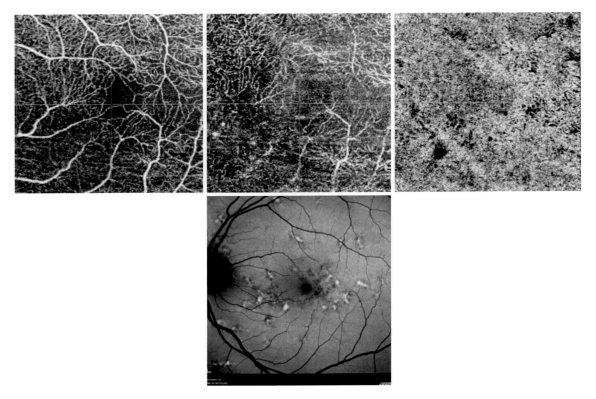

Fig. 1. Stargardt's disease in a 27-year-old patient. Top left: Optical coherence tomography angiography (OCT-A) of the superficial capillary plexus, showing limited rarefaction of the vessel. Top center: OCT-A of the deep capillary plexus, revealing attenuation and loss of capillaries. Top right: OCT-A of the choriocapillaris, with dark areas associated with the masking effects of the flecks and decreased vascular density. Bottom: Short-wavelength fundus autofluorescence of the same case.

amplitude-decorrelation angiography algorithm. This instrument has an A-scan rate of 100,000 scans per second, wavelength scanning light centered on 1,050 nm and an in-depth resolution of 2.6 μm (digital). Each OCT-A scan (3 × 3, 4.5 × 4.5 or 6 × 6 mm) contains 256 B-scans (each B-scan contains 256 A-scans). To image the motion of scattering particles (erythrocytes), 4 sequential OCT raster scans are performed and are repeated at the same location on the retina (assisted by eye tracking).

Dystrophies with Prevalent Central Involvement
Many dystrophies are characterized by prevalent central involvement, most frequently including Stargardt's disease, Best vitelliform macular dystrophy, pattern dystrophy of the retinal pigment epithelium,

cone-rod and cone dystrophies, and central areolar choroidal dystrophy. All of these disorders typically show alterations at the level of the outer retina, leading to the progressive development of macular atrophy. OCT-A can reveal a relatively normal superficial capillary plexus, whereas the deep capillary plexus shows attenuation of the retinal vessels, along with some areas of perifoveal capillary loss, especially in eyes affected by Stargardt's disease (fig. 1, 2). In particular, the extent of deep retinal plexus abnormalities often exceeds that of atrophic changes, as visualized on short-wavelength fundus autofluorescence (fig. 1, 2), suggesting that the deep capillary structures undergo a different degenerative process with respect to photoreceptor-retinal pigment epithelial cells. The superficial and deep plexuses are generally

Battaglia Parodi · Pierro · Gagliardi · Lattanzio · Querques · Bandello

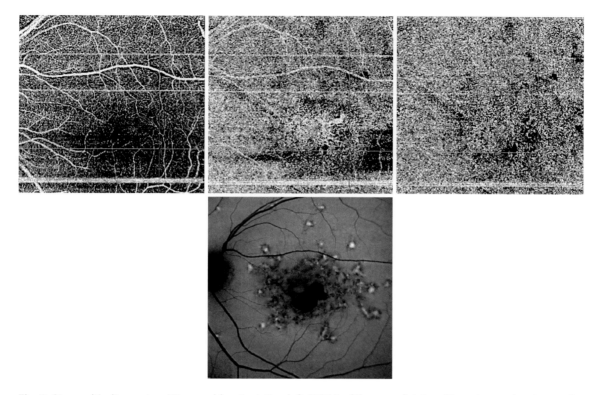

Fig. 2. Stargardt's disease in a 32-year-old patient. Top left: OCT-A of the superficial capillary plexus, showing a relatively normal vascular pattern. Top center: OCT-A of the deep capillary plexus, with attenuation and rarefaction of the capillaries. Top right: OCT-A of the choriocapillaris, disclosing darker areas corresponding to flecks and reduced vascular density. Bottom: Short-wavelength fundus autofluorescence of the same case.

normal in eyes affected by pattern dystrophies (fig. 3). However, the choriocapillaris layer can also contain some regions of attenuation and density reduction (fig. 1–3). It is of interest that both flecks and pigment deposition can be visualized at the choriocapillaris level as darker lesions, perfectly corresponding to alterations detectable on biomicroscopic and color examinations (fig. 1–3), and they are likely related to masking effects due to material deposition. OCT-A findings are also variably altered in patients with Best vitelliform macular dystrophy, showing similar features (fig. 4).

Dystrophies with Prevalent Peripheral Involvement
Retinitis pigmentosa, choroideremia, and gyrate atrophy are the most important dystrophy subtypes with prevalent peripheral involvement. OCT-A is

generally aimed at assessment of the central macular area (3 × 3 and 6 × 6) rather than the periphery. Thus, most analyses are performed on the central region to identify features that could be correlated with pathogenetic and prognostic characteristics. Indeed, patchy areas of limited perfusion can be detected within the macular area analyzed. In particular, the deep plexus may appear to be more involved, showing attenuation of the capillary vessels with reduced density in the whole macular area (fig. 5, 6). In some cases, the border between the residual normal retina and the affected retina is not completely delineated on OCT-A, suggestive of a more complex vascular impairment. In addition, the choriocapillaris shows remarkably abnormal flow (fig. 5, 6). Analysis of vascular patterns in patients affected by choroideremia is more complex, as they are only identifiable in the

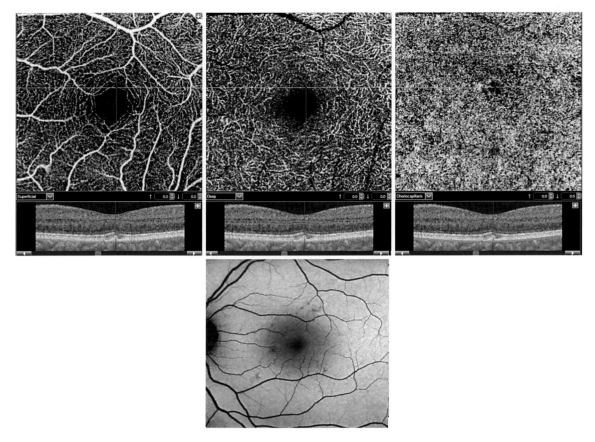

Fig. 3. Adult-onset vitelliform macular dystrophy in a 51-year-old female. Top left: OCT-A of the superficial capillary plexus, showing a normal appearance. Top center: OCT-A of the deep capillary plexus with a normal vascular pattern. Top right: OCT-A of the choriocapillaris, characterized by darker foveal areas corresponding to pigment deposition and an irregular vascular density. Bottom: Short-wavelength fundus autofluorescence of the same case.

spared macular area. In particular, although the superficial plexus is only slightly impaired, the deep capillary plexus and choriocapillaris are clearly altered (fig. 7).

Discussion

OCT-A represents a pioneering noninvasive imaging technique that can provide new information regarding retinal and choroidal vascular flow. In particular, OCT-A can reveal vascular dysfunction, and such information can be useful in the stage classification of each dystrophy, and it can theoretically be correlated with the long-term progression of the disease, allowing for the additional assessment of the treatment response.

The most important vascular layers can be separately analyzed, and future attempts will be made to quantify both retinal and choroidal blood flow, especially when patchy areas of impaired perfusion are identified.

Battaglia Parodi · Pierro · Gagliardi · Lattanzio · Querques · Bandello

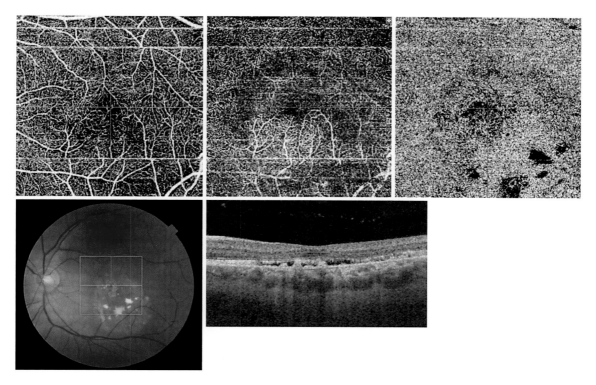

Fig. 4. Best vitelliform macular dystrophy in a 46-year-old male. Top left: OCT-A of a relatively normal superficial capillary plexus. Top center: OCT-A of the deep capillary plexus with an extremely abnormal vascular pattern. Top right: OCT-A of the choriocapillaris, disclosing several darker areas corresponding to vitelliform material deposition and an abnormal vascular density. Bottom left: Color image of the same cases. Bottom right: Optical coherence tomography of the same case, showing partial reabsorption of the vitelliform material.

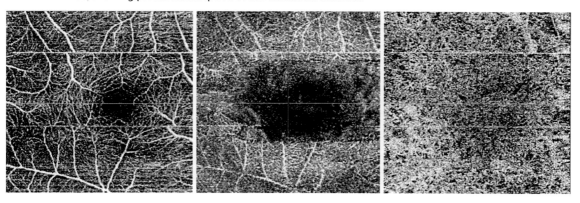

Fig. 5. Retinitis pigmentosa in a 58-year-old male. Left: OCT-A of the superficial capillary plexus with an almost regular pattern. Center: OCT-A of the partially detectable deep capillary plexus. In the residual deep plexus, attenuation and loss of capillaries are visible. Right: OCT-A of the choriocapillaris, disclosing many areas with absence of vascular flow.

Fig. 6. Retinitis pigmentosa in a 66-year-old male. Left: OCT-A of an almost normal superficial capillary plexus. Center: OCT-A of the partially visible deep capillary plexus, revealing attenuation and loss of capillaries. Right: OCT-A of the choriocapillaris, showing a reduced vascular density. *(For figure see next page.)*

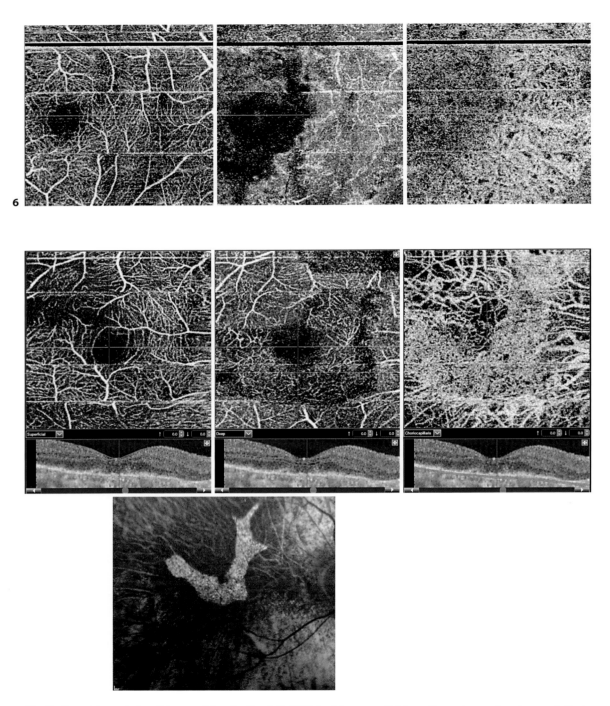

Fig. 7. Choroideremia in a 34-year-old male. Top left: OCT-A of the superficial capillary plexus, showing a relatively spared pattern. Top center: OCT-A of the deep capillary plexus, with identification at the level of the residual macular region. Top right: OCT-A of the choriocapillaris, which is visible just in the residual central retina, showing attenuation. Bottom: Short-wavelength fundus autofluorescence of the same case.

The detection of vascular abnormalities in dystrophies on OCT-A may indicate that the pathogenesis and natural evolution of each disorder are also affected by the vascular supply. Thus, our observations can have direct therapeutic implications for the future practical management of retino-choroidal dystrophies.

References

1 Jia Y, Tan O, Tokayer J, et al: Split-spectrum amplitude-decorrelation angiography with optical coherence tomography. Opt Express 2012;20:4710–4725.

2 Choi W, Mohler KJ, Potsai B, et al: Choriocapillaris and choroidal microvasculature imagin with ultrahigh speed OCT angiography. PLoS One 2013;8:E81499.

3 Jia Y, Bailey SJ, Hwang TS, et al: Quantitative optical coherence tomography angiography of vascular abnormalities in the living human eye. Proc Natl Acad Sci U S A 2015;112:E2395–E2402.

Maurizio Battaglia Parodi
Department of Ophthalmology, Ospedale San Raffaele
Via Olgettina 61
IT–20132 Milan (Italy)
E-Mail battagliaparodi.maurizio@hsr.it

Bandello F, Souied EH, Querques G (eds): OCT Angiography in Retinal and Macular Diseases.
Dev Ophthalmol. Basel, Karger, 2016, vol 56, pp 166–173 (DOI: 10.1159/000442809)

Swept-Source Optical Coherence Tomography Angiography of Paediatric Macular Diseases

Paulo E. Stanga[a–c] · Alessandro Papayannis[a, b] · Emmanouil Tsamis[a–c] ·
Katarzyna Chwiejczak[a, b] · Francesco Stringa[a] · Assad Jalil[a, b] · Tim Cole[d] ·
Susmito Biswas[a–c]

[a]Manchester Vision Regeneration (MVR) Lab at Manchester Royal Eye Hospital & NIHR/Wellcome Trust Manchester CRF,
Manchester, [b]Manchester Royal Eye Hospital, Central Manchester University Hospitals NHS Foundation Trust, Manchester
Academic Health Science Centre, Manchester, [c]Institute of Human Development, Faculty of Medical and Human Sciences,
University of Manchester, Manchester, and [d]Topcon (GB) Ltd., Newbury, UK

Abstract

Purpose: To describe the optical coherence tomography (OCT) angiography (OCTA) features of paediatric macular pathologies. **Methods:** Retrospective serial case reports of patients who underwent routine clinical examination and OCTA of the posterior pole using both a DRI OCT Atlantis prototype and Triton Swept-Source OCT. When considered necessary, imaging was performed using Optos wide-field imaging or another non-invasive imaging system. The findings were compared with the current literature. **Results:** Three cases with X-linked retinoschisis, 2 with epiretinal membrane, 1 with Best disease and 2 with Coats disease are fully illustrated. **Conclusion:** OCTA is an effective, non-invasive imaging technique that can offer additional information regarding the morphologies and vascular characteristics of macular lesions in paediatric ophthalmology. Because of the rarity and characteristics of many paediatric macular pathologies, further multi-centric research is required with regard to the utilisation and features of OCTA imaging.

© 2016 S. Karger AG, Basel

Introduction

Indirect ophthalmoscopy remains the first and basic technique used to visualize the fundus in children. With the advent of new imaging modalities, physicians have received a rich armoury of techniques, facilitating the diagnosis of retinal diseases. Nevertheless, retinal imaging in the paediatric population remains a challenge, as it requires cooperation, and for this reason, it has to be performed under anaesthesia in many cases.

Until recently, the only way to extract information about the retinal and choroidal vasculature has been the implementation of fundus fluorescein angiography (FFA) and indocyanine green angiography, respectively. To facilitate imaging in children, a RetCam (Clarity Medical Systems, Pleasenton, Calif., USA) contact fundus camera, also supporting FFA imaging, has been introduced [1]. Still, it is difficult to obtain images during early phases [2].

Nonetheless, intravenous administration of contrast material is an **invasive procedure**, and possible adverse reactions have been reported in 3–20% of cases, according to different studies [3]. It may also require **general anaesthesia**, which involves risks and requires appropriate equipment, medications and personnel trained in paediatric resuscitation [4]. Furthermore, insufficient data are available to exclude a potentially negative influence of anaesthesia on neurodevelopment [5, 6].

To reduce any risk related to intravenous injection, fluorescein can be administered orally, with adverse reactions observed in 1–2% of patients; however, nausea and vomiting are not uncommon, and high-intensity early-phase images cannot be readily obtained [7, 8].

For the purposes of paediatric clinics, where procedures need to be non-invasive and ideally performed with portable devices, a hand-held optical coherence tomography (OCT) device has been developed. It provides results comparable to those of conventional chin-rest spectral domain OCT and allows for rapid data acquisition [9], but it lacks the ability to depict vasculature.

Optical coherence tomography angiography (OCTA) can be considered a promising new technique in ophthalmic paediatrics, giving hope that at least some of the current problems associated with imaging of the retinal and choroidal vessels in children may be solved. Its safety, non-invasiveness and short acquisition time may be beneficial for examination of the posterior fundus in children who are old enough to cooperate and maintain a chin-rest position. Hence, the limitations and risks of FFA can be avoided.

In this chapter, we describe OCTA features in serial and single paediatric cases. The rarity of some of the conditions and the consequent lack of case series data imply that a critical perspective should be adopted for interpretation of these case reports.

X-Linked Retinoschisis

X-linked retinoschisis is an X-linked recessive disorder caused by a mutation in the RS1 gene encoding retinoschisin, and it occurs almost exclusively in young males [10]. This condition leads to early-onset bilateral visual loss due to foveal schisis from the splitting of the inner retinal layers, mainly within the inner nuclear layer. Other possible sight-threatening complications are as follows: retinal detachment, vitreous haemorrhage or intraretinal haemorrhage within a schisis cavity [11, 12]. Vascular changes similar to Coats disease have been described in X-linked retinoschisis [11].

We analysed OCT angiograms of the right eye of a 9-year-old boy (with a history of complicated retinal detachment and subsequent enucleation of the left eye) and of both eyes of two children who were 16 and 17 years old (Cases 1–3). All of these cases presented with petaloid non-reflective areas in the macular zone located predominantly inside of the deep neurovascular plexus. In both the superficial and deep neurovascular plexuses, in all cases, there was evidence of perifoveal microvascular alterations similar to teleangectasias. Analysis of the choriocapillaris revealed areas of hypo- and hyper-reflectivity that were not associated with any evident aspect of a vascular alteration but could be attributed to alterations in OCTA signal due to a shadow effect or to retinal pigment epithelium irregularities, respectively (fig. 1) [13].

Fig. 1. (Cases 1–3). From left to right, optical coherence tomography (OCT) angiography (OCTA) images of the outer, inner and choriocapillaris vascular plexuses and OCTA B-scans of 5 eyes. Three male children with X-linked retinoschisis. Top row, right eye of a 9-year-old boy (after enucleation of the left eye); second to fifth row, images of both eyes of two children aged 16 and 17 years, respectively. The red arrows point to some hyper-reflective microvascular alterations similar to teleangectasias that are evident in both the superficial and deep neurovascular layers.

(For figure see next page.)

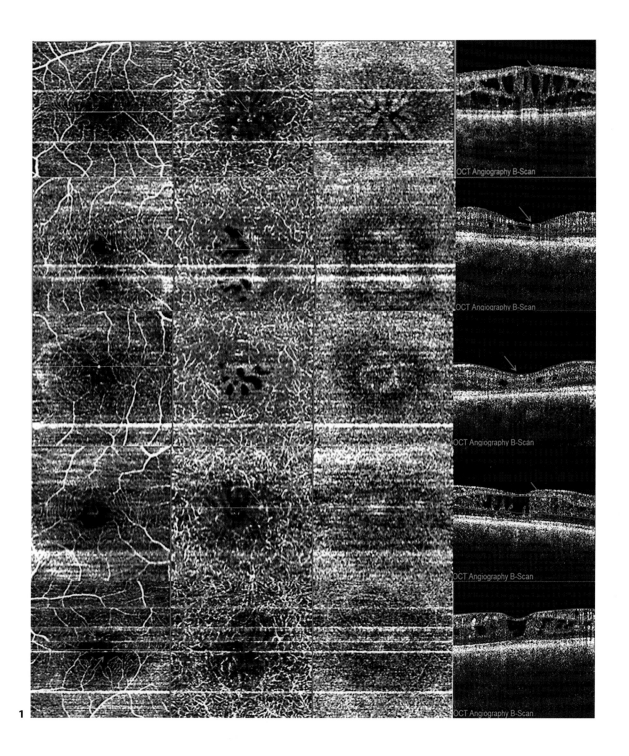

1

Stanga · Papayannis · Tsamis · Chwiejczak · Stringa · Jalil · Cole · Biswas

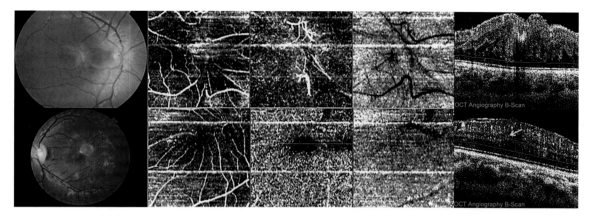

Fig. 2. (Cases 4–5). Two cases of a 14-year-old girl (images on the bottom) and an 11-year-old boy (images on the top) with idiopathic epiretinal membranes in the left and right eyes, respectively. From left to the right: colour fundus images, outer and inner vascular networks and choriocapillaris OCT angiograms and B-scans. The red arrows indicate the major epiretinal vessels that were dislocated in the depth of the retinal layers, invading the foveal avascular zone, and their shadow effects on choroidal OCT angiograms. The yellow arrow highlights the erroneous automated segmentation due to massive thickening of the neuroepithelium.

Epiretinal Membrane

Epiretinal membrane (ERM) is a rare finding in children and is usually secondary to another condition, such as traumatism, inflammation, or a tumour, but it can also occur in the absence of any underlying condition [14]. It leads to decreased visual acuity and metamorphopsia.

Two cases of a 14-year-old girl and an 11-year-old boy with idiopathic ERM in the left and right eyes, respectively, are illustrated (Cases 4–5). In both cases, the massive anatomic disruption associated with abnormal thickening of the retinal layers due to the ERM resulted in many errors in automated segmentation of the retinal layers. This led to difficult and erroneous segmentation in many scans that could not be adjusted in the absence of a manual segmentation option. In the second case, an interesting finding was the presence of 'conglomeration/phagocytosis' of the epiretinal vessels inside of the deep vascular plexus due to profound disruption of the architecture of the retinal layers, with the subsequent presence of this massive hyper-reflective vascular structure

in the respective OCTA images. The abnormal delocalization of big vessels towards the depth of the retina and the macular area led to the presence of non-reflective lines on the choroidal OCT angiograms that represented 'negative' projections of the major retinal vessels created by their shadow effects (fig. 2).

Best Disease (Best Vitelliform Macular Dystrophy)

Best disease is the second most common dystrophy of the macula. It is inherited in an autosomal dominant manner and is caused by a mutation in the bestrophin gene. It is characterized by abnormal accumulation of lipofuscin at the level of the retinal pigment epithelium [10, 15]. The evolution of Best disease can be separated into 5 stages, from an asymptomatic stage to a scarring stage. One of the complications of this pathology is choroidal neovascularization (CNV), which is described in the most advanced stage of the disease and is associated with a poor visual outcome [16].

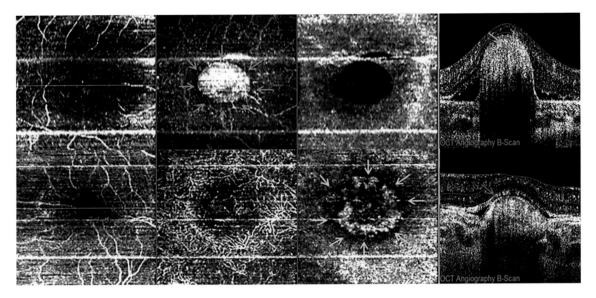

Fig. 3. (Case 6). OCT angiograms of both eyes of a 16-year-old boy with Best disease and a history of choroidal neovascularization (CNV) in the right eye (top row images). From left to right, superficial, deep and choriocapillaris vascular network OCT angiograms and corresponding B-scans. The green arrows indicate an intense homogeneous hyper-reflective circular lesion in the macular area due to a CNV fibrovascular scar. The orange arrow in the B-scan image highlights the CNV scar tissue, which is reaching the inner plexiform layer/inner nuclear layer delimited border, disrupting all underlying layers. The yellow arrows show an inhomogeneous hyper-reflective circular lesion in the choriocapillaris angiogram due to deposits of lipofuscin material. The red arrow indicates the preserved retinal pigment epithelium and inner segment/outer segment bands.

We illustrate the case of a 16-year-old boy with Best disease with a history of subretinal neovascularization in the right eye (Case 6). In both eyes, the anatomic disruption was associated with abnormal thickening of the retinal layers; this thickening was due to CNV in the right eye and to the presence of lipofuscin material in the left eye. As a consequence, automated segmentation of the deep retinal layer and the choriocapillaris was poor. Both eyes had a relatively preserved aspect of the superficial neurovascular plexus.

In the right eye with the CNV scar, there was an intense homogeneous hyper-reflective circular lesion in the macular area due to a non-vascular decorrelation signal. As highlighted in the B-scan image, the CNV invaded the deep neurovascular layer to the inner plexiform layer/inner nuclear layer delimited border.

In the left eye, the deep neurovascular plexus was preserved, and an inhomogeneous hyper-reflective circular lesion was evident on OCT angiograms of the choriocapillaris due to the presence of deposits of lipofuscin material, also generating a non-vascular decorrelation signal [17] (fig. 3).

Coats Disease

Coats disease is an idiopathic, progressive retinal vascular disorder that is probably associated with the NDP gene. It is characterized by retinal telangiectasia and multiple saccular aneurysmal dilations in the retinal vasculature, leading to intraretinal and subretinal exudation with consequent exudative retinal detachment [18, 19]. Neovascular changes resembling retinal angiomatous pro-

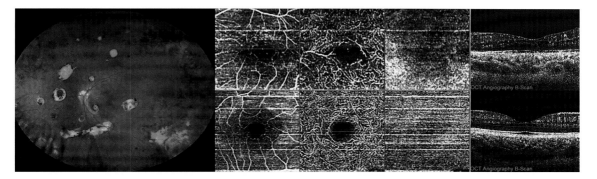

Fig. 4. (Case 7). Optos wide-field colour fundus image (left image) and OCT angiograms (DRI OCT-1 Atlantis, Topcon) of superficial, deep and choriocapillaris vascular plexuses and the corresponding OCTA B-scan images (from left to right). The top row shows the left eye of a 15-year-old boy after treatment with transcleral drainage of the fluid and anti-VEGF injection. The red arrows indicate rarefaction of the superficial and especially of the deep vascular plexus. The bottom row shows OCT angiograms and a B-scan of the right eye, showing no significant vascular alterations.

liferation and macular chorioretinal anastomoses have also been described. Some authors have used the term 'macular fibrosis' to describe lesions generated either from chronic subretinal exudation or retinal vascular anastomoses resulting in fibrosis [18].

The cases of two boys with Coats disease in the left and right eyes, respectively, the first of whom was 15 years of age (Case 7) and the second of whom was 6 years of age (Case 8), are described below. The first case had been treated with transcleral drainage of the fluid and anti-VEGF injection [19], while the second case had received laser treatment of only the peripheral lesions due to the presence of a macular fibrotic lesion at baseline.

In the first case, there was evident rarefaction of the superficial and especially of the deep vascular plexus with a preserved choriocapillaris. On the contrary, the second case showed complete disruption of all retinal layers, preventing any standardised segmentation due to the absence of reference points. For this reason, the segmentation in this case was performed manually to evaluate the characteristics of four adjacent levels across the fibrotic tissue, from the inner limiting membrane to the choriocapillaris,

which had different reflectivity intensities on B-scan. The results of the described segmentation analysis of the fibrotic lesion highlighted the presence of a dense hyper-reflective fibrovascular structure in the first three layers due to a non-vascular decorrelation signal, ending with a fourth deeper choroidal layer with non-reflective characteristics due to a shadow effect of the overlying tissue [20].

Furthermore, the presence of such a big scar is associated with loss of fixation, resulting in low-quality decentred images during the acquisition process in the absence of eye-tracking technology (fig. 4, 5).

Conclusions

Although OCTA has been demonstrated to be an encouraging new technique for the assessment of challenging paediatric ophthalmic cases, there are limitations that must be overcome in the future. First, the implementation of currently available OCTA devices with eye-tracking technology is crucial for poorly cooperative patients, such as children. Moreover, the portability of OCTA, possibly achieved by the development of hand-

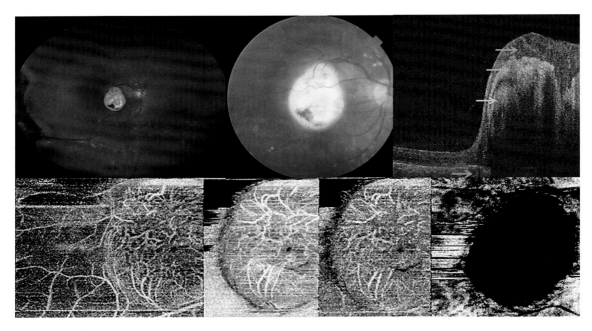

Fig. 5. (Case 8). Six-year-old boy with a fibrotic macular lesion due to Coats disease who was treated with peripheral laser only at the peripheral lesions. Top row, left to right, Optos wide-field colour fundus, posterior pole colour fundus and OCT B-scan images. Bottom row, from left to right, OCT angiograms (with DRI OCT Triton, Topcon) of the four adjacent levels across the fibrotic tissue with different reflectivity intensities on B-scan, with labelling from the inner limiting membrane to the choriocapillaris using four different-coloured arrows, respectively.

held devices, can be an essential advancement allowing for the examination of patients of toddler age. Due to the rarity of most of these paediatric conditions, further multi-centric research needs to be undertaken to enhance our knowledge regarding the application of this non-invasive technique and to enable the rapid establishment of a normative database. When standardised, OCTA can be used as a routine examination, thereby reducing the risks associated with the use of invasive techniques on patients in the paediatric age group.

References

1 Kim JW, Ngai LK, Sadda S, Murakami Y, Lee DK: Retcam fluorescein angiography findings in eyes with advanced retinoblastoma. Br J Ophthalmol 2014;98: 1666–1671.

2 Tsui I, Franco-Cardenas V, Hubschman JP, Schwartz SD: Pediatric retinal conditions imaged by ultra wide field fluorescein angiography. Ophthalmic Surg Lasers Imaging 2013;44:59–67.

3 Kalogeromitros DC, Makris MP, Aggelides XS, Mellios AI, Giannoula FC, Sideri KA, Rouvas AA, Theodossiadis PG: Allergy skin testing in predicting adverse reactions to fluorescein: a prospective clinical study. Acta Ophthalmol 2011;89:480–483.

4 Hildebrand GD: Imaging the fundus; in Hoyt CS, Taylor D (eds): Pediatric Ophthalmology and Strabismus, ed 4. Edinburgh: Saunders/Elsevier Ltd. 2013, pp 63–70.

5 Mann GE, Kahana M: The uncomfortable reality. We simply do not know if general anesthesia negatively impacts the neurocognitive development of our small children. Int J Pediatr Otorhinolaryngol 2015;79:1379–1381.

6 Lee JH, Zhang J, Wei L, Yu SP: Neurodevelopmental implications of the general anesthesia in neonate and infants. Exp Neurol 2015;272:50–60.

7   Brockow K, Sánchez-Borges M: Hyper-sensitivity to contrast media and dyes. Immunol Allergy Clin North Am 2014; 34:547–564.

8   Watson AP, Rosen ES: Oral fluorescein angiography: reassessment of its relative safety and evaluation of optimum conditions with use of capsules. Br J Ophthalmol 1990;74:458–461.

9   Mallipatna A, Vinekar A, Jayadev C, Dabir S, Sivakumar M, Krishnan N, Mehta P, Berendschot T, Yadav NK: The use of handheld spectral domain optical coherence tomography in pediatric ophthalmology practice: our experience of 975 infants and children. Indian J Ophthalmol 2015;63:586–593.

10 Nentwich M, Guenther R: Hereditary retinal eye diseases in childhood and youth affecting the central retina. Oman J Ophthalmol 2013;6(suppl 1):S18–S25.

11 Kim DY, Mukai S: X-linked juvenile retinoschisis (XLRS): a review of genotype-phenotype relationships. Semin Ophthalmol 2013;28:392–396.

12 Gregori NZ, Berrocal AM, Gregori G, Murray TG, Knighton RW, Flynn HW Jr, Dubovy S, Puliafito CA, Rosenfeld PJ: Macular spectral-domain optical coherence tomography in patients with X linked retinoschisis. Br J Ophthalmol 2009;93:373–378.

13 Stringa F, Papayannis A, Tsamis E, Chwiejczak K, Biswas S, Jalil A, Stanga PE: Optical coherence tomography angiography: a new imaging approach for the assessment of macular changes in X-linked juvenile retinoschisis. Seattle, 2016 ARVO Annual Meeting, Research: A Vision of Hope, May 1–5, 2016.

14 Bonnin S, Metge F, Guez A: Long-term outcome of epiretinal membrane surgery in young children. Retina DOI: 10.1097/IAE.0000000000000732.

15 Ferrara DC, Costa RA, Tsang S, Calucci D, Jorge R, Freund KB: Multimodal fundus imaging in Best vitelliform macular dystrophy. Graefes Arch Clin Exp Ophthalmol 2010;248:1377–1386.

16 Chung MM, Oh KT, Streb LM, Kimura AE, Stone EM: Visual outcome following subretinal hemorrhage in best disease. Retina 2001;21:575–580.

17 Lumbroso B, Huang D, Fujimoto JG, Jia Y, Rispoli M: Clinical Guide to Angio-OCT: Non Invasive, Dyeless OCT Angiography. New Delhi, Jaypee Brothers Medical Publishers, 2015.

18 Battaglia Parodi M, Zucchiatti I, Fasce F, Cascavilla ML, Cicinelli MV, Bandello F: Dome-shaped macula associated with Best vitelliform macular dystrophy. Eur J Ophthalmol 2015;25:180–181.

19 Stanga PE, Jaberansari H, Bindra MS, Gil-Martinez M, Biswas S: Transscleral drainage of subretinal fluid, anti-vascular endothelial growth factor, and wide-field imaging-guided laser in coats exudative retinal detachment. Retina 2016; 36:156–162.

20 Chwiejczak K, Papayannis A, Stringa F, Tsamis E, Biswas S, Jalil A, Stanga PE: Optical coherence tomography angiography imaging and ultra wide-field multi-wavelength imaging after transscleral drainage of subretinal fluid, anti-vascular endothelial growth factor, and wide-field imaging-guided laser in coats' exudative retinal detachment. Seattle, 2016 ARVO Annual Meeting, Research: A Vision of Hope, May 1–5, 2016.

Paulo E. Stanga
Manchester Vision Regeneration (MVR) Lab
Research Office, Purple Zone, MRI
Central Manchester University Hospitals NHS
Foundation Trust
Oxford Road
Manchester M13 9WL (UK)
E-Mail Paulo.Stanga@cmft.nhs.uk

Bandello F, Souied EH, Querques G (eds): OCT Angiography in Retinal and Macular Diseases.
Dev Ophthalmol. Basel, Karger, 2016, vol 56, pp 174–180 (DOI: 10.1159/000442810)

Optical Coherence Tomography Angiography of Miscellaneous Retinal Disease

Luisa Pierro · Maurizio Battaglia Parodi · Alessandro Rabiolo · Ugo Introini · Giuseppe Querques · Francesco Bandello

Department of Ophthalmology, University Vita-Salute, San Raffaele Scientific Institute, Milan, Italy

Abstract

In this chapter, we illustrate different clinical scenarios using swept-source optical coherence tomography angiography (OCTA, Triton, Topcon, Inc., Tokyo, Japan). The instrument is based on a long wavelength scanning light (1,050 nm) that can better penetrate the deeper ocular layers, such as the choroid and sclera. Our aim was to show how OCTA can be used to study the eye vascular network in a novel and innovative fashion. We have demonstrated that a specific disease can involve one or more layers; conversely, the same layer may be affected by different ocular pathologies. Moreover, we would like to stress that knowledge of disease pathophysiology is fundamental, and thus, we have focused our attention on the layer(s) most involved in each pathological condition. In some miscellaneous cases, the swept-source OCTA findings have corroborated with conventional imaging data (i.e. fundus photography, B-scan ultrasonography, fluorangiography and indocyanine green angiography), thus leading us to the proper diagnosis.

In this chapter, we illustrate different clinical scenarios using swept-source optical coherence tomography angiography (SS-OCTA, Triton, Topcon, Inc., Tokyo, Japan). The instrument is based on a long wavelength scanning light (1,050 nm) that can better penetrate the deeper ocular layers, such as the choroid and sclera. Moreover, SS-OCT allows for the clear visualization of both the vitreous and choroid in a single scan, free from artifacts.

In some miscellaneous cases, SS-OCTA findings have corroborated with conventional imaging data (i.e. fundus photography, B-scan ultrasonography, fluorangiography and indocyanine green angiography), thus leading us to the proper diagnosis. SS-OCTA may also allow to better understand of the pathophysiologies of different retinal diseases.

The manuscript is not under simultaneous consideration by any other publication.

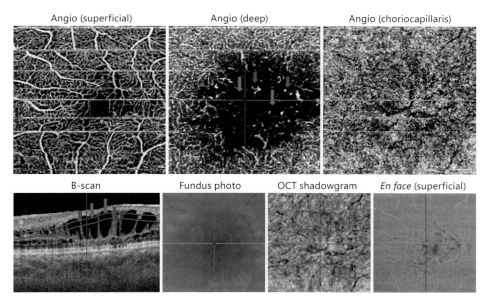

Fig. 1. Case 1. **X-linked retinoschisis.** Left eye of a 9-year-old male patient afflicted with X-linked retinoschisis. B-scan shows the typical appearance of retinoschisis macular edema, characterized by multiple thin intraretinal columns. The deep capillary plexus (corresponding to the tissue between the two green parallel lines on the B-scan image) appears to be the most affected vascular layer. In contrast with macular edema by other causes, the black pseudocystic areas (red arrows) are much larger and are partially interspersed with residual vascular tissue, which appears as fragmented white spots (green arrows). The differences from other types of macular edema are probably due to different pathogenetic mechanisms, as X-linked retinoschisis is related to a reduction in retinoschisin, implying retinal layer adhesion defects.

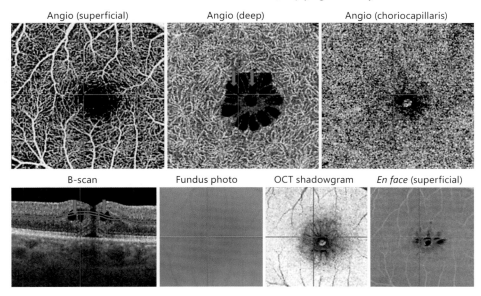

Fig. 2. Case 2. **Full-thickness macular hole.** Right eye of a 63-year-old male patient affected by a full-thickness macular hole (small stage, International Vitreomacular Traction Study Group Classification). The deep capillary plexus (green lines on B-scan image) is the most affected. Swept-source optical coherence tomography angiography (SS-OCTA) shows a wheel-like central lesion, with cystic spaces at the hole boundaries (red arrows). The surrounding network is denser compared to normal eyes. We hypothesize that steepening of the macular hole edges may determine this vascular engorgement.

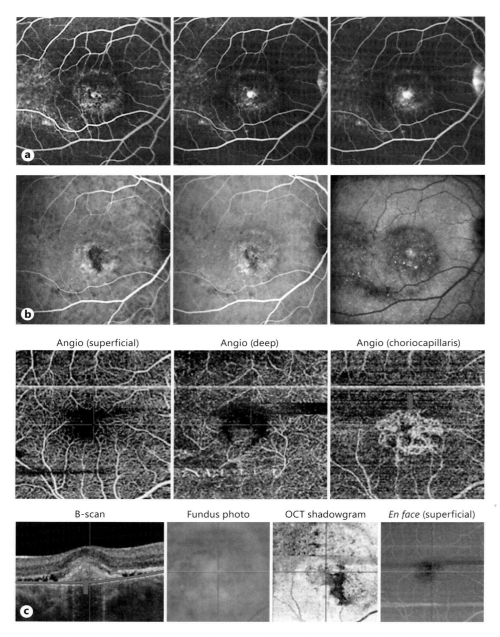

Angio (superficial)   Angio (deep)   Angio (choriocapillaris)

B-scan   Fundus photo   OCT shadowgram   *En face* (superficial)

Fig. 3. Case 3. **Best disease.** Right eye of a 12-year-old female patient affected with Best disease. Interestingly, fluorescein angiography (**a**) and indocyanine green angiography (**b**) were fairly suggestive of active choroidal neovascularization. SS-OCTA (**c**) reveals a vascular tuft (green arrows) in the choriocapillaris (green lines on B-scan image), consistent with active neovascularization.

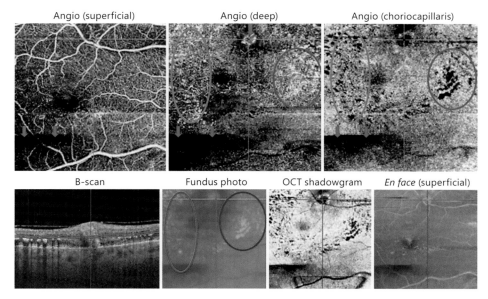

Fig. 4. Case 4. **Retinal macroaneurysm.** Right eye of a 75-year-old male patient with retinal macroaneurysm along the superior vascular arcade. At the deep segmented layer (green lines on B-scan image), SS-OCTA scan reveals a small hyper-reflective circular lesion (red arrow) surrounded by an irregular vascular network. The diffuse white hyper-reflective spots correspond to the highest areas of exudate (blue circles), which appear as several black spots in the choriocapillary layer due to a shadow effect. The black areas visible (green arrows) at the bottoms of all images are consistent with hemorrhage migration.

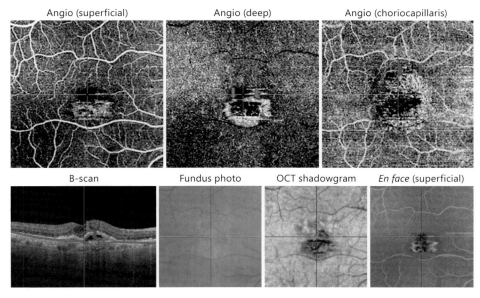

Fig. 5. Case 5. **Drusenoid pigment epithelial detachment (PED).** Right eye of a 77-year-old female patient affected by drusenoid PED. The patient had been previously treated for choroidal neovascularization in the fellow eye. At the segmented deep layer, SS-OCTA reveals a circular hyper-reflective area corresponding with the highest area of PED (red arrows) at B-scan. In the choriocapillary layer (green lines on B-scan image), arched vascular tissue is present (green arrows) along the PED, suggestive of neovascularization beneath the PED area.

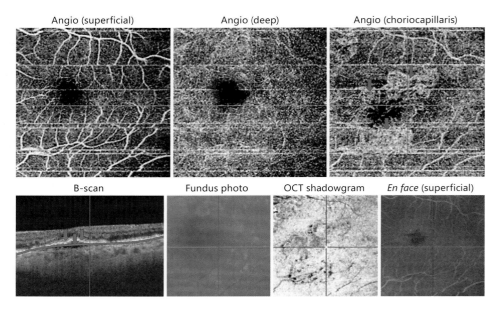

Angio (superficial)   Angio (deep)   Angio (choriocapillaris)

B-scan   Fundus photo   OCT shadowgram   *En face* (superficial)

Fig. 6. Case 6. **Retinal pigment epithelium (RPE) irregularity.** Left eye of a 73-year-old female patient with RPE irregularity. The B-scan image shows irregular alteration of the RPE, which appears slightly elevated (red arrows). At the choriocapillary layer (green lines on B-scan image), SS-OCTA shows a large irregular vascular network (green arrows), suggestive of a quiescent neovascular lesion.

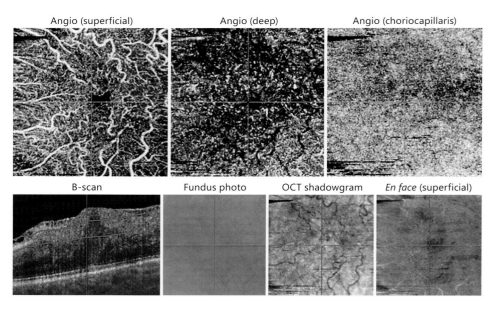

Angio (superficial)   Angio (deep)   Angio (choriocapillaris)

B-scan   Fundus photo   OCT shadowgram   *En face* (superficial)

Fig. 7. Case 7. **Epiretinal membrane.** Left eye of a 71-year-old male patient suffering from epiretinal membrane. The B-scan image shows an epiretinal membrane adherent to the inner retinal layers causing tractional intraretinal edema. The superficial plexus (green lines on B-scan image) is the most affected, showing vessel stretching and tortuosity due to membrane traction. In addition, some vascular abnormalities are evident in the deep plexus.

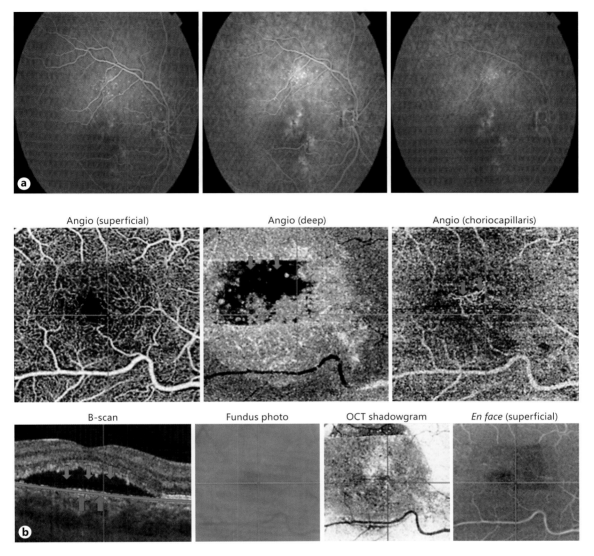

Fig. 8. Case 8. **Central serous chorioretinopathy.** Right eye of a 45-year-old male patient affected by central serous chorioretinopathy. The B-scan image shows neuroretinal detachment consistent with central serous chorioretinopathy (red arrows). Although fluorescein angiography (**a**) revealed only broad areas of granular hyperfluorescence, SS-OCTA (**b**) shows branching neovessels (green arrows) in the choriocapillaris (green lines on B-scan image).

Disclosure Statement

The authors declare that there are no conflicts of interest.

References

1 Unterhuber A, Povazay B, Hermann B, Sattmann H, Chavez-Pirson A, Drexler W: In vivo retinal optical coherence tomography at 1,040 nm – enhanced penetration into the choroid. Opt Express 2005;13:3252–3258.

2 Choi W, Mohler KJ, Potsaid B, Lu CD, Liu JJ, Jayaraman V, Cable AE, Duker JS, Huber R, Fujimoto JG: Choriocapillaris and choroidal microvasculature imaging with ultrahigh speed OCT angiography. PLoS One 2013;8:e81499.

3 Bonini Filho MA, De Carlo TE, Ferrara D, Adhi M, Baumal CR, Witkin AJ, Reichel E, Duker JS, Waheed NK: Association of choroidal neovascularization and central serous chorioretinopathy with optical coherence tomography angiography. JAMA Ophthalmol 2015;133: 899–906.

4 De Carlo TE, Bonini Filho MA, Chin AT, Adhi M, Ferrara D, Baumal CR, Witkin AJ, Reichel E, Duker JS, Waheed NK: Spectral-domain optical coherence tomography angiography of choroidal neovascularization. Ophthalmology 2015;122:1228–1238.

5 Inoue M, Balaratnasingam C, Freund KB: Optical coherence tomography angiography of polypoidal choroidal vasculopathy and polypoidal choroidal neovascularization. Retina 2015;35: 2265–2274.

Luisa Pierro
Department of Ophthalmology, University Vita-Salute
San Raffaele Scientific Institute, Via Olgettina 60
IT–20132 Milan (Italy)
E-Mail pierro.luisa@hsr.it

Subject Index